D1479733

Continuous Hemofiltration

Contributions to Nephrology

Vol. 93

KARGER

Basel · München · Paris · London · New York · New Delhi · Bangkok · Singapore · Tokyo · Sydney

2nd International Conference on Continuous Hemofiltration,
Baden/Austria, September 10–11, 1990

Continuous Hemofiltration

Volume Editors
H.G. Sieberth, *H. Mann*, Aachen
H.K. Stummvoll, Linz

77 figures and 72 tables, 1991

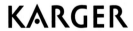

Basel · München · Paris · London · New York · New Delhi · Bangkok · Singapore · Tokyo · Sydney

Contributions to Nephrology

Library of Congress Cataloging-in-Publication Data
    International Conference on Continuous Hemofiltration (2nd: 1990: Baden, Austria)
    Continuous hemofiltration/2nd International Conference on Continuous Hemofiltration, Baden/Austria, September 10–11, 1990;
    volume editors, H.G. Sieberth, H. Mann, H.K. Stummvoll.
    (Contributions to nephrology: vol. 93)
    Includes bibliographical references and index.
    (alk. paper)
    1. Continuous arterovenous hemofiltration – Congresses. 2. Multiple organ failure – Treatment – Congresses. 3. Acute renal failure – Treatment – Congresses. I. Sieberth (Heinz Günter) II. Mann, H. (Helmut) III. Stummvoll, H.K. ´ IV. Title. V. Series: Contributions to nephrology; v. 93. [DNLM: 1. Antibiotics – pharmakokinetics – congresses. 2. Hemofiltration – congresses. 3. Kidney Failure, Acute – physiopathology – congresses. 4. Kidney Failure, Acute – therapy. 5. Multiple Organ Failure – congresses. W1 CO77BUN v. 93/WJ 342 159003c 1990]
    RC901.7.H47156 1990   617.4´61059 dc20
    ISBN–3–8055–5375–7

Bibliographic Indices
    This publication is listed in bibliographic services, including Current Contents ᴿ and Index Medicus.

© Copyright 1991 by S. Karger AG, P.O. Box, CH-4009 Basel (Switzerland)
    Printed in Switzerland on acid-free paper by Thür AG Offsetdruck, Pratteln
    ISBN 3–8055–5375–7

Contents

Contents

Cardiac and Pulmonary Diseases

Pharmacokinetics

Technical Aspects of Solute Transport

Anticoagulation

Miscellaneous

Contents

Preface

The mortality rate of acute renal failure dropped from more than 80% to 30% after intermittent hemodialysis was introduced to the treatment of acute renal failure. Two decades later, until 1970, the mortality rose again up to 70%. Rising mortality developed parallel to the establishment of intensive care units. The progress in the field of intensive care created a lot of critically ill patients reaching the state of acute renal failure, who would have died in earlier times before reaching acute renal failure because of the severity of their underlying disease. We know today that the reason for this is not acute renal failure, but multi-organ failure. The death rate is rising with the number of organ failures. The failure of four vital organs is followed by a death rate of nearly 100%, independent of the fact whether acute renal failure is included or not.

While the first Symposium on continuous hemofiltration held in Aachen in 1984 was devoted more to techniques, parenteral nutrition and single-organ failure, this time multi-organ failure is the main subject of discussion. Also, our panel discussion dealt with this problem. First of all, during this discussion we have to raise the question: Is multi-organ failure only the sum of different organ failures, or is there a common basic origin which perhaps can be explained biochemically?

The second main topic of this Symposium was the therapy of acute renal and multi-organ failure. This again raises the question: Do we have a real chance to reduce the still high mortality rate of our patients with multi-organ failure?

On this problem larger groups of patients were presented at the Symposium. Again, controlled surveys permitting a statistically proved comparison between continuous and intermittent treatment cannot be submitted. But even if continuous treatment is more effective than intermittent treatment, death rate will still remain high. To diminish the high mortality rate in patients with multi-organ failure we have to improve the function not only of the kidney but also of the other organs, and/or we have to eliminate the still unknown common mechanism of multi-organ failure.

We hope that continuous hemofiltration and the Symposium were steps in this direction.

H.G. Sieberth

Sieberth HG, Mann H, Stummvoll HK (eds): Continuous Hemofiltration.
Contrib Nephrol. Basel, Karger, 1991, vol 93, pp 1–12

Continuous versus Intermittent Treatment: Clinical Results in Acute Renal Failure

H. Kierdorf

Medizinische Klinik II (Direktor: Prof. *H.G. Sieberth*), RWTH Aachen, FRG

In 1977, Kramer et al. [1] first reported continuous treatment for acute renal failure (ARF). They had developed continuous arteriovenous hemofiltration (CAVH). This system represented the first form of therapy to enable continuous artificial substitution of one organ system. CAVH was very rapidly adopted as a simple technique which could be used anywhere, even in departments with a lack of experience of treating ARF. However, the method frequently proved inadequate for hemodynamically unstable patients with hypercatabolic renal failure.

Since the beginning of the 1980s, a number of other continuous treatment methods have been developed, like continuous arteriovenous hemodialysis (CAVHD), in some cases combined with plasma separation (CAVHDP), or like pump-driven venovenous methods (CVVH or CVVHD). Their common feature is a higher effectiveness in the control of azotemia also in hypercatabolic patients [2, 3].

Clinical or experimental studies comparing these new continuous forms of treatment in controlled prospective studies with the established intermittent hemodialysis treatment are missing. The question of whether these new forms of treatment for ARF are generally superior to intermittent hemodialysis, or whether some groups of patients may profit from it, can currently be answered only be reference to theoretical advantages, by investigations of some single factors and by a few retrospective studies which compare the clinical outcome of continuous and intermittent therapy. This question seems to be of great interest, because since 1950 the mortality of ARF has risen continuously and is currently almost 70% [4]. In the literature, the rise in mortality for ARF is attributed to two main causes [5–9]: (1) A reduction of cases with uncomplicated ARF, partly due to improved shock prophylaxis. (2) An increase in multiorgan failure (MOF) resulting from extremely severe illnesses, accidents or operations, also affecting older patients. Owing to the improvements in all areas of intensive care medicine, ARF now affects many patients who would formerly have died before the condition could occur.

Table 1. Advantages (A) and disadvantages (D) of continuous and intermittent treatment

Continuous treatment		Intermittent treatment	
A	hemodynamic stability	(D	hemodynamic instability)
A	fluid elimination	D	rapid fluid and solute shift
A	membrane compatibility	D	membrane incompatibility
D	continuous anticoagulation	A	mobilization, single needle
D	immobilization, arterial puncture	A	bicarbonate-buffered dialysate
		A	higher efficiency

Advantages and Disadvantages of Continuous and Intermittent Treatment

Theoretical advantages and disadvantages of both types of treatment have been discussed by numerous authors. Some of these individual factors have also been examined in clinical studies (table 1) [4, 8, 10, 11].

Hemodynamics. Hemodynamic instability, especially in patients with MOF, is one of the main indications for the use of continuous treatment in ARF. Some authors could show that hemodialysis treatment cannot be carried out on approximately 10% of all patients with ARF due to hemodynamic instability [12, 13]. Paganini et al. [14] demonstrated in 1984 that 23 patients of their collective, for whom neither dialysis nor isolated intermittent mechanical ultrafiltration was possible, could be treated by continuous filtration. Conversely, Mukau and Latimer [15] reported in 1988 no patients untreatable with hemodialysis in a group with surgically associated MOF. This study relied, however, on bicarbonate hemodialysis, for which a significantly higher hemodynamic stability had been demonstrated by recent authors [16, 17].

In the absence of specific clinical studies to establish whether there are patients who cannot be treated by intermittent methods, one can only reflect the clinical impression of virtually all nephrologists, that intermittent treatment has to be interrupted in roughly 5–10% of all cases of ARF, even where bicarbonate hemodialysis is employed. This agrees with the results of a retrospective study of Mauritz et al. [18] comparing continuous and intermittent methods, in which significantly more episodes of sudden hypotension in the dialysis treatment group are described. Several authors have recently demonstrated a positive long-term effect of continuous hemofiltration on the hemodynamic situation of the patients [2, 10, 14, 19, 20]. Lauer et al. [19] could show by right heart catheter measurements, a significant rise in the cardiac index in continuous treated patients after a mean total ultrafiltration of 7 liters. Mean arterial blood pressure was unchanged. The improvement in myocardial function is in part caused by the change in preload, leading to a more optimal point on the Starling curve. It is not yet clear whether identical negative balance in intermittent dialysis avoids this convincing cardiac effect. Continuous hemolfiltration has been shown to decrease Apache II scores and to increase arterial blood pressure significantly [21]. In contrast to these and nearly all other authors, Kohen et al. [22] concluded in a retrospective analysis in 1985, based on the data of only 3 patients, that the number of hypotensive crises in intermittent hemodialysis treatment was significantly higher than in CAVH, but that, by comparison with the effective elimination of urea, the relative frequency of hypotensive incidents during hemodialysis was significantly lower.

Fluid Elimination, Parenteral Nutrition. Kohen et al. [22] are also the only authors to report more effective and less stressful fluid elimination in intermittent hemodialysis. In contrast to this opinion in a review of the literature, the undisputed advantage of continuous treatment is the avoidance of electrolyte fluctuation and fluid imbalances [1–4, 11, 20, 23]. There is no limitation of fluid intake in continuous treatment forms, enabling parenteral nutrition to be adapted to the needs of the patients with ARF. Especially in anuric patients, despite daily hemodialysis, hyperhydration frequently occurs during intermittent treatment, due to parenteral feeding, blood compounds and drug infusions. Recent studies during the last years imply that particularly MOF patients benefit from the use of continuous treatment, because the unlimited supply of energy and protein eliminates the effect of malnutrition on the mortality of these critically ill patients [24–28]. When conventional dialysis treatment is used, there is regularly a risk of insufficient nutrition due to limitations on fluid intake. In a prospective study we could demonstrate in 1986 a significant reduction in protein catabolism with adapted amino acid intake for a group of 30 patients with ARF (fig. 1) [29]. Slow continuous correction of electrolytes and fluid balance significantly reduces cerebral alterations in continuous treated patients, because rapid sodium and fluid shifts in intermittent hemodialysis could be demonstrated to be responsible for the cerebral side effects of hemodialysis therapy [30]. The increase in intracranial pressure in intermittent treatment can be avoided using continuous hemofiltration, possibly also contributing to the reduction of cerebral side effects when continuous methods are used [31, 32].

Membrane Incompatibility. Complement activation and an increase in leukocytes and thrombocytes is described for intermittent hemodialysis

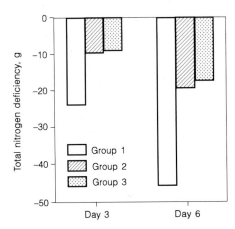

	Group 1	Group 2	Group 3
Days of treatment	73	65	85
Amino acid dose, g/kg bw	0.7	1.5	1.74
Ultrafiltrate, liters/day	18.2	18.9	19.4
Nitrogen excretion, g/day	15.4	17.9	19.1
Nitrogen balance, g/day	−8.1	−3.4	−3.2

Fig. 1. Nitrogen balance in ARF during CVVH treatment related to different amounts of amino acid intake [29].

[33]. In various studies in recent years, Hörl's working group demonstrated different intensities for this activation dependent on the dialysator's material [34–36]. In 1983, Böhler et al. [37] demonstrated that this activation does not occur when polysulfone or polyacrylnitrite (PAN) membranes are used either in continuous or in intermittent hemofiltration. This appears to represent an advantage, particularly for MOF patients, because the leukocyte drop combined with complement activation may namely be responsible for the hypoxemia which regularly occurs at the beginning of hemodialysis [38]. This hypoxemia may be an expression of leukocyte sequestration in the pulmonary circulation [38]. A question remains open in this context, whether the use of continuous hemodialysis does not likewise lead to corresponding activation of the systems, since a clear distinction has so far been established only between filtration and dialysis and not between continuous and intermittent treatment.

Anticoagulation. Apart from a few exceptions in individual cases, continuous treatment methods require continuous anticoagulation. Intermittent hemodialysis has the advantage of requiring anticoagulation, if at all, over a limited period only [39]. Various authors agree that the average heparin requirement of patients is roughly 500 U/h [3, 11, 40–42]. In patients with a higher bleeding risk, this dose can be significantly reduced with an acceptable filter running time [40]. A lower anticoagulant requirement in continuous dialysis was mentioned which has not yet been

Table 2. Bicarbonate-buffered replacement fluid for continuous treatment (values are mmol/l)

	Golper, 1985 [8]	Kierdorf
Na	147	140
Cl	115	110
HCO$_3$	36	34
K	0	0
Ca	1.2	1.75
Mg	0.7	0.5
Glucose	6.7	5.6

documented by clinical studies. The theoretical background may be the higher blood viscosity in the venous line in continuous hemofiltration, which can lead to earlier filter occlusion. Anticoagulation can be completely dispensed in certain continuously treated patients as described for CAVHD with a filtration time of approximately 10 h (max. 30 h) [40]. Alternative anticoagulants such as prostacyclin and its stable analogues may also reduce the disadvantages of continuous treatment as opposed to intermittent hemodialysis [42].

Arterial Punctures, Immobilization. Intermittent hemodialysis can be carried out via a single central catheter. CAVH and CAVHD require an arterial access, either in the form of a catheter in the arteria femoralis or as a Scribner shunt [43]. This implies the risk of arterial puncture or disconnection bleeding, which had been described in personal communications by a number of working groups for CAVH, and the patients need to be immobilized. This risk does not apply using pump-driven methods such as CVVH or CVVHD. Pump-drive filtration or dialysis has been demonstrated adequately with one double-lumen Shaldon catheter, eliminating this disadvantage of continuous treatment compared to intermittent hemodialysis [44, 45].

Substitution Fluid: Bicarbonate vs. Lactate Buffer. Hyperlactatemia has been noted to be a disadvantage of continuous filtration and dialysis. This may be caused by the lactate buffer in the substitution and dialysis fluid [46]. As early as 1985, the possibility of bicarbonate-buffered substitution in CAVH, avoiding the metabolic disadvantages of lactate buffering, had been pointed out [8]. The solution is compared in table 2 to a bicarbonate-buffered solution we have been using for 2 years (Schiwa & Co., Glandorf, FRG).

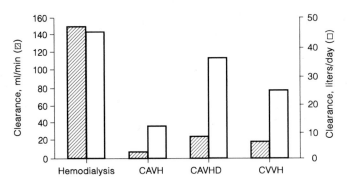

Fig. 2. Efficiency of different forms of treatment. Results for CAVH, CAVHD and CVVH are averaged for all studies cited in this paper, daily clearance for hemodialysis was calculated for a daily 4-hour treatment.

Efficiency of the Different Forms of Treatment. Essential criterion for the effectiveness of different methods of extracorporeal treatment is the control of azotemia. Intermittent hemodialysis is superior to all other methods in terms of its efficiency per unit time. Depending on blood and dialysate flow and on the type of filter employed, urea clearances of between 120 and 180 ml/min can be achieved. This is equivalent to a daily urea clearance of up to 50 liters, if a 4-hour daily treatment is used (fig. 2.)

The clearance achieved with continuous methods is comparatively low. Data collected from all cited studies in this paper indicate an average clearance of 5–10 ml/min for CAVH, of 15–30 ml/min for CAVHD and of 12–20 ml/min for CVVH. Comparing daily clearance CAVHD and CVVH obtain more favorable results owing to their 24-hour treatment, though normally without achieving the clearances attained by intermittent dialysis. The effectiveness of both methods can, however, be improved if the clinical situation demands either by increasing dialysate flow rate or by increasing daily filtration rate. A comparison of studies of continuous treated patients (table 3) restricted to patients with at least one additional vital function disturbance (60–70% of the cases with MOF) clearly demonstrates that CAVH in most cases is inadequate as the sole therapy for azotemia in hemodynamically unstable hypercatabolic patients with ARF [3, 8, 10, 20, 23, 41, 47]. By comparison, the intensified continuous therapies, i.e. CAVHD, CVVH or CVVHD, regularly achieve a reduction in urea and creatinine concentration [2, 3, 20, 21, 40, 41, 48–54]. Various comparative studies have also documented significantly greater effectiveness for CAVHD and CVVH as opposed to CAVH in MOF patients [3, 17, 55–59].

Table 3. Efficiency of different forms of continuous treatment

Authors	Treatment	Clearance ml/min	Ultrafiltration l/day	Q_D ml/h	Urea
Kramer et al., 1980 [23]	CAVH	–	7.5	–	↑
Weisse et al., 1989 [47]	CAVH	–	8–10	–	→ (↑)
Stevens et al., 1988 [20]	CAVHD	14–22	?	1,000	↓
Canaud et al., 1988 [41]	CVVH	–	11.6	–	↘

Table 4. Comparison of CAVH and CVVH in the treatment of MOF [57]

	CAVH (n = 24)	CVVH (n = 28)
Days of treatment (mean)	12.4	16.2*
Ultrafiltration, liters/day (mean)	13.1	21.8*
Filter running time (mean)	26	32.4*
Additional intermittent hemodialysis (in relation to CAVH/CVVH day)	0.1	0*
Urea pretreatment/after 72 h, mmol/l	480/390	462/285*
Creatinine pretreatment/after 72 h, μmol/l	38.5/31	39.2/21*

*$p < 0.001$.

Maher et al. [56] demonstrated the superiority of CAVHD to CAVH for his patients, significantly improving clearance with CAVHD by increasing the dialysis flow rate from 1 to 1.5 liters/h at a constant blood flow, while a further increase to 2 liters/h achieved only a slight additional increase in clearance. Gibney et al. [49] demonstrated for CAVHD that an effective reduction in urea concentration can be achieved even at a lower dialysate flow rate (600–900 ml/h). Their patients had higher ultrafiltration rates compared to other studies. In a comparative retrospective study, Mauritz et al. [18] found adequate control of urea in intermittent dialysis and CVVH, whereas CAVH was insufficient for controlling azotemia. We could also demonstrate the distinct superiority of CVVH as against CAVH. Apart from significantly lower serum urea and creatinine concentrations, a particularly impressive finding was that patients in the CVVH group required no additional intermittent hemodialysis and were less catabolic (table 4) [57].

Outcome in ARF and MOF: Influence of the
Different Forms of Treatment?

Unlike ARF in the 1950s, today in most of the cases it is no longer an isolated organ function disturbance but part of a MOF. MOF patients have an exceptionally poor prognosis, with a mortality of 80–100%. The mortality increases with the number of vital function disturbances, both in patients primarily affected by ARF [4] and in those MOF patients whose renal function is primarily adequate [58]. Until now the question whether the selected form of treatment can influence the development and the progress of a MOF or can decisively reduce patient mortality is not yet answered. In most patients the progress of MOF cannot be influenced, despite intensive medication, surgical and/or extracorporeal treatment.

As mentioned above, prospective studies comparing the outcome in ARF correlated to different forms of treatment are not present. Three relevant retrospective studies uniquely compare intermittent hemodialysis with continuous treatment. Barzilay et al. [59, 60] demonstrated a statistically significant increase in the survival rate of MOF patients treated by continuous methods as compared to conventional therapy. Surprisingly, the MOF patients with the highest chance of survival were those treated by a combined method using CAVHD and plasma separation, unfortunately not explained in greater detail. A criticism of this study is that the information on the MOF and on the patient data are very small. For example, it is not noted whether any of the patients suffered from a renal failure or, if so, to what extent [60].

Mauritz et al. [18] compared hemodialysis, CAVH and CVVH. This detailed study showed no statistical significance for one of the three groups in terms of their survival rate, but indicated a clear trend in favor of a

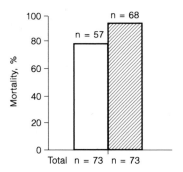

Fig. 3. Mortality in ARF. Comparison of intermittent hemodialysis (▨) and CVVH (▢).

higher survival rate for patients treated with pump-driven continuous filtration. In addition, the authors described a statistically higher renal recovery rate in the CVVH group.

We carried out a retrospective study comparing 73 patients treated by continuous hemofiltration from 1986 to 1988 with 73 patients treated by intermittent hemodialysis. These 73 intermittently treated patients were randomized retrospectively from a total of 243 patients, so that the group was comparable to the continuous-treatment group in terms of age, sex and number of vital function disturbances. There was a significantly lower mortality in the CVVH group, only 57 of the 73 patients died, as compared to 68 in the group of 73 dialyzed patients (fig. 3). In addition, there was a correlation between mortality and the number of vital function disturbances in both groups.

Despite the fact that in retrospective analyses continuous methods appear to reduce mortality in critically ill patients with ARF, randomized prospective studies are necessary to demonstrate clearly the benefit compared to intermittent forms of treatment.

References

1   Kramer P, Wigger W, Rieger J, Matthaei D, Scheler F: Arteriovenous haemofiltration: A new and simple method for treatment of overhydrated patients resistant to diuretics. Klin Wochenschr 1977;55:1121–1122.

2   Geronemus R, Schneider N: Continuous arteriovenous haemodialysis: A new modality for treatment of acute renal failure. Trans Am Soc Artif Intern Organs 1984;30:610–613.

3   Van Geelen JA, Vincent HH, Schalekamp MADH: Continuous arteriovenous haemofiltration and haemodiafiltration in acute renal failure. Nephrol Dial Transplant 1988;2:181–186.

4   Sieberth HG, Kierdorf H: Is continuous haemofiltration superior to intermittent dialysis and haemofiltration treatment; in Hörl WH, Schollmeyer PJ (eds): New Perspectives in Haemodialysis, Peritoneal Dialysis, Arteriovenous Haemofiltration and Plasmapheresis. New York, Plenum Press, 1990 pp 181–192.

5   Butkus DE: Persistent high mortality in acute renal failure. Arch Intern Med 1983;2:209–212.

6   Kindler J, Frisch J, Meister M, Grittmann G, Genn I, Sieberth HG: Akutes Nierenversagen beim Multiorganversagen. Intensivmedizin 1986;23:241–246.

7   Cameron JS: Acute renal failure in the intensive care unit. Intensive Care Med 1986;12:64–70.

8   Golper TA: Continuous arteriovenous haemofiltration in acute renal failure. Am J Kidney Dis 1985;6:373–386.

9   Lazarus JM: Acute renal failure. Intensive Care Med 1986;12:61–63.

10   Favre H: Haemodialysis, peritoneal dialysis or continuous extracorporeal epuration in acute renal failure patients. Contrib Nephrol. Basel, Karger, 1989, vol 71, pp 100–103,

11   Bartlett RH, Bosch J, Geronemus R, Paganini E, Ronco C, Swartz R: Continuous arteriovenous hemofiltration for acute renal failure. Trans Am Soc Artif Intern Organs 1988;34:67–77.

12   Keshaviah P, Shapiro FL: A critical examination of dialysis-induced hypotension. Am
      J Kidney Dis 1982;2:290–293.
13   Van Stone JC, Bauer J, Carey J: The effect of dialysate sodium concentration on body
      fluid compartment volume, plasma renin activity and plasma aldosterone concentration
      in chronic haemodialysis patients. Am J Kidney Dis 1982;2:58–62.
14   Paganini EP, O'Hara P, Nakamoto S: Slow continuous ultrafiltration in haemodialysis
      resistant oliguric acute renal failure patients. Trans Am Soc Artif Intern Organs
      1984;30:173–178.
15   Mukau L, Latimer RG: Acute haemodialysis in the surgical intensive care unit. Am
      Surg 1988;54:548–552.
16   Huyghebaert MF, Dhainaut JF, Monsallier JF, Schlemmer B: Bicarbonate haemodialysis
      of patients with acute renal failure and severe sepsis. Crit Care Med 1985;12:840–843.
17   Leunissen KML, Hoorntje SJ, Fiers HA, Dekkers WT, Mulder AW: Acetate versus
      bicarbonate haemodialysis in critically ill patients. Nephron 1986;42:145–151.
18   Mauritz W, Sporn P, Schindler I, Zadrobilek E, Roth E, Appel W: Acute renal failure
      in abdominal infection. Comparison of haemodialysis and continuous arteriovenous
      haemofiltration. Anästh Intensivther Notfallmed 1986;21:212–217.
19   Lauer A, Alvis R, Avram M: Haemodynamic consequences of continuous arteriovenous
      haemofiltration. Am J Kidney Dis 1988;12:110–115.
20   Stevens PE, Riley B, Davies SP, Gower PE, Brown EA, Kox W: Continuous arteri-
      ovenous haemodialysis in critically ill patients. Lancet 1988;ii:150–152.
21   Wendon J, Smithies M, Sheppard M, Bullen K, Tinker J, Bihari D: Continuous high
      volume veno-venous haemofiltration in acute renal failure. Intensive Care Med
      1989;15:358–363.
22   Kohen JA, Whitley KY, Kjellstrand CM: Continuous arteriovenous haemofiltration: A
      comparison with haemodialysis in acute renal failure. Trans Am Soc Artif Intern Organs
      1985;31:169–173.
23   Kramer P, Kaufhold G, Grone HJ, Wigger W, Rieger J, Mathaei D, Stokke T,
      Burchardi H, Scheler F: Management of anuric intensive care patients with arteri-
      ovenous haemofiltration. Int J Artif Organs 1980;3:225–230.
24   Bartlett RH, Mault JR, Deckert RE, Palmer J, Swartz RD, Port FK: Continuous
      arteriovenous haemofiltration: Improved survival in surgical acute renal failure? Surgery
      1986;100:400–408.
25   Bartlett RH: Energy metabolism in acute renal failure; in Sieberth HG, Mann H (eds):
      Continuous Arteriovenous Hemofiltration (CAVH). Basel, Karger, 1985, pp 194–203.
26   Mault JR, Bartlett RH, Deckert RE, Clark SF, Swartz RD: Starvation: A major
      contributing factor to mortality in acute renal failure. Trans Am Soc Artif Intern
      Organs 1983;29:390–394.
27   Mault JR, Kresowik TF, Deckert RE, Arnoldi DK, Swartz RD, Barlett RH: Continu-
      ous arteriovenous haemofiltration: The answer to starvation in acute renal failure. Trans
      Am Soc Artif Intern Organs 1984;30:203.
28   Abel RM, Beck CH, Abbott WM, Ryan JA, Barnett GO, Fischer JE: Improved survival
      from acute renal failure after treatment with intravenous essential L-amino acids and
      glucose. N Engl J Med 1973;288;695–698.
29   Kierdorf H, Kindler J, Sieberth HG: Nitrogen balance in patients with acute renal
      failure treated by continous arteriovenous haemofiltration. Nephrol Dial Transplant
      1986;1:72.
30   Kleeman CR: CNS manifestations of disordered salt and water balance. Hosp Pract
      1979;14:59–74.
31   Davenport A, Will EJ, Losowsky MS: Rebound surges of intracranial pressure as a

consequence of forced ultrafiltration used to control intracranial pressure in patients with severe hepatorenal failure. Am J Kidney Dis 1989;14:516–519.

32 Bertrand YM, Hermat A, Mahieu P, Roels J: Intracranial pressure changes in patients with head trauma during haemodialysis. Intensive Care Med 1983;9:321–323.

33 Jakob AI, Gavellas G, Zarco R, Perez G, Bourgoignie JJ: Leukopenia, Hypoxemia and complement function with different haemodialysis membranes. Kidney Int 1980;18:505–509.

34 Hörl WH, Schaefer RM, Heidland A: Effect of different dialyzers on proteinases and proteinase inhibitors during haemodialysis. Am J Nephrol 1985;5:320–326.

35 Hörl WH, Riegel W, Schollmyer P, Rautenberg W, Neumann S: Different complement and granulocyte activation in patients dialyzed with PMMA dialyzers. Clin Nephrol 1986;25:304–307.

36 Haag-Weber M, Schollmeyer P, Hörl WH: Granulocyte activation during haemodialysis in the absence of complement activation: inhibition by calcium channel blockers. Eur J Clin Invest 1988;18:380–385.

37 Böhler J, Kramer P, Götze O, Schwartz P, Scheler F: Leucocyte counts and complement activation during pump-driven and arteriovenous haemofiltration. Contrib Nephrol Basel, Karger, 1983, vol 36, pp 15–25.

38 Craddock PR, Fehr J, Brigham KL, Kronenberg RS, Jakob HS: Complement and leukocyte-mediated pulmonary dysfunction in haemodialysis. N Engl J Med 1977;296:769–774.

39 Casati S, Moia M, Graziani G, Cantaluppi A, Citterio A, Mannucci PM, Ponticelli C: Haemodialysis without anticoagulants: Efficiency and haemostatic aspects. Clin Nephrol 1984;21:102–105.

40 Geronemus RP: Slow continuous haemodialysis, Trans Am Soc Artif Intern Organs 1988;34:59–60.

41 Canaud G, Carred LJ, Christol JP, Aubas S, Beraud JJ, Mion C: Pump-assisted continuous venovenous haemofiltration for treating acute uremia. Kidney Int 1988;33(suppl 24):S154–S156.

42 Zobel G, Ring E, Müller W: Continuous arteriovenous haemofiltration in premature infants. Crit Care Med 1989;17:534–536.

43 Keshaviah PR: Technical aspects of continuous and intermittent therapies. Trans Am Soc Artif Intern Organs 1988;34:61–62.

44 Bregman H, Miller K, Berry L: Minimum performance standards for double-lumen subclavian cannulas for haemodialysis. Trans Am Soc Artif Intern Organs 1986;32:500–502.

45 Kierdorf H, Kindler J, Heintz B, Maurin N, Sieberth HG: Continuous haemofiltration in cases of acute renal failure with double-lumen Shaldon catheters. Kidney Int 1990;37:1175.

46 Reynolds HN, Belzberg H, Connelly J: Hyperlactemia in patients undergoing continuous arteriovenous haemofiltration with dialysis. Crit Care Med 1990;18:582.

47 Weisse L, Danielson BG, Wikstroem B, Hedstrand U, Wahlberg J: Continuous arteriovenous haemofiltration in the treatment of 100 critically ill patients with acute renal failure: report on clinical outcome and nutritional aspects. Clin Nephrol 1989;31:184–189.

48 Chanard J, Milcent T, Toupance O, Melin JP, Roujouleh H, Lavaud S: Ultrafiltration pump-assisted continuous arteriovenous haemofiltration (CAVH). Kidney Int 1988;33(suppl 24):S157–S158.

49 Gibney RT, Sollery DE, Lefebvre RE, Sharun CJ, Chan P: Continuous arteriovenous haemodialysis: an alternative therapy for acute renal failure associated with critical illness. Can Med Assoc J 1988;139:861–866.

50   Paganini EP: Slow continuous haemofiltration and slow continuous ultrafiltration. Trans Am Soc Artif Intern Organs 1988;35:63–66.
51   Schneider NS, Geronemus RP: Continuous arteriovenous haemodialysis. Kidney Int 1988;33(suppl 24):159–162.
52   Tam PY, Huraib S, Mahan B, LeBlanc D, Lunsky CA, Holtzer C, Doyle CE, Vas SI, Uldall PR: Slow continuous haemodialysis for the management of complicated acute renal failure in an intensive care unit. Clin Nephrol 1988;30:79–85.
53   Tighe MR, Hall CL: Continuous arteriovenous haemodialysis in critically ill patients. Lancet 1988;ii:458–459.
54   Alrabi AA, Danielson BG, Wikstroem B: Continuous dialysis in acute renal failure. Scand J Urol Nephrol 1990;24:1–5.
55   Raja R, Kramer M, Goldstein S, Caruana R, Lerner A: Comparison of continuous arteriovenous haemofiltration and continuous arteriovenous dialysis in critically ill patients. Trans Am Soc Artif Intern Organs 1986;32:435–436.
56   Maher ER, Hart L, Levy D, Scoble JE, Baillod RA, Sweny P, Varghese Z, Moorhead JF: Comparison of continuous arteriovenous haemofiltration and haemodialysis in acute renal failure. Lancet 1988;i:129.
57   Kierdorf H, Kindler J, Maurin N, Glöckner WM, Heintz B, Sieberth HG: Acute renal failure: Comparison between arteriovenous (CAVH) and venovenous (CVVH) haemofiltration. Abstr XIth Int Congr Nephrology, Tokyo 1990, p 147.
58   Knaus WA, Draper EA, Douglas MS, Wagner DP, Zimmerman JE: Prognosis in acute organ-system failure. Ann Surg 1985;112:685–693.
59   Barzilay E, Berlot G, Kessler D, Geber D: More on acute renal failure in the intensive care unit. Intensive Care Med 1989;15:478.
60   Barzilay E, Kessler D, Berlot G, Gullo A, Geber D, Zeev IB: Use of extracorporeal supportive techniques as additional treatment for septic-induced multiple organ failure patients. Crit Care Med 1989;17:634–637.

Dr. H. Kierdorf, Department of Internal Medicine II, Pauwelsstrasse 30,
D–W–5100 Aachen (FRG)

Sieberth HG, Mann H, Stummvoll HK (eds): Continuous Hemofiltration.
Contrib Nephrol. Basel, Karger, 1991, vol 93, pp 13-16

Long-Term Experience with Continuous Renal Replacement Therapy in Intensive-Care Unit Acute Renal Failure

Cindy Bosworth, Emil P. Paganini, Frank Cosentino, Robert J. Heyka

The Cleveland Clinic Foundation, Cleveland, Ohio, USA

An average of 160 intensive-care unit (ICU) patients per year are seen by the nephrology service at the Cleveland Clinic Foundation. Of these, 66–78% have required some form of dialytic intervention. This patient population is tracked through a registry containing demographic and daily data on each patient. Using this data base, 3 years of therapy (1986, 1988, 1989) were reviewed (n = 320 patients). This allowed us to describe and compare the patient profile of those who were treated with continuous (C) therapy, intermittent hemodialysis (I) and those treated with a combination of intermittent/continuous (IC) therapies.

Patients and Methods

Patients. The patient profile consisted of 61% males with a mean age of 60 ± 15.7. 75% were postoperative cases with 29.5% of this group having undergone coronary artery bypass (CABG) surgery. 58% of the patients had a serum creatinine >1.4 mg/dl on admission but were not on dialytic support. In addition, 94% were oliguric (urine output <500 cc/day) at the start of therapy.

29.7% were treated with C, 27.3% with IC and 43% with I therapy.

Description of Therapy. On I therapy, hemodialysis was done approximately every other day using a cuprophane membrane (Allegro). The average treatment was 4 h with removal of 2 litres of fluid. Access was predominantly through a double-lumen (Medcomp) femoral venous catheter. Subclavian access was used in $<10\%$ of the patients. The average mean arterial pressure (MAP) of these patients was 85 mm Hg.

Within the group on C therapy, 8% were treated with slow continuous ultrafiltration exclusively, 7% were treated with continuous arteriovenous hemodialysis (CAVHD) exclusively and 45% were on continuous arteriovenous hemofiltration (CAVH) exclusively. The remaining 40% were treated with combinations of the three continuous types during their course of therapy. C therapy was maintained for 6.52 ± 6.25 consecutive days with a maximum range of 63 days. The hemofilters used were polyamide (Gambro/CAVH) or polyacrylonitrile (Asahi CAVHD). A bicarbonate-based electrolyte solution was used as replacement solution for CAVH. The solution was delivered post-hemofilter with an average of 10 litres of fluid exchanged during the 24 h. For CAVHD, a peritoneal dialysate solution

(Dineal, Baxter, 1.5%) was used at an average dialysate flow of 14 litres/24 h. On CAVH and CAVHD average net fluid removal was 1 liter/day. Access was exclusively through single-lumen arterial and venous femoral catheters (Medcomp).

Results

Lower MAPs were noted in the patients on C therapy (69.5 mm Hg with blood pressure support required 97% of the time). The average MAP in the IC group was 78.9 mm Hg. The results of the levels of blood urea nitrogen and serum creatinine are shown in table 1.

Patients were followed with APACHE II scores [1]. These were calculated twice in each patient, on admission to ICU (A_1) and also at time of renal consult (A_2). The scores calculated on CABG surgery patients were reported separately because of the possibility of error with this application of the score. The differences in the two scores were reviewed and an A_2/A_1 ratio calculated. This ratio was >1 in the C group, <1 in the I group and 1 or >1 in the IC group, indicating that those patients who became worse during their ICU stay were treated with C therapy.

Multiorgan dysfunction (3 or more organs) has been seen to increase from 69 to 79% over the last 2 years. In addition to renal failure, those system dysfunctions most frequently occurring in the patient group who did not survive included: pulmonary failure (mechanical ventilation required) = 100%; gastrointestinal (hyperbilirubinemia >2.0) = 74.4%, and cardiovascular (systolic blood pressure <90) = 68.9%. Sepsis as a cause of death increased from 23.7 to 50.7%.

Hospital survival of the ICU patients was for 1986: I = 19%, C = 19%, IC = 24%; for 1988: I = 54%, C = 21%, IC = 32%, and for 1989: I = 46%, C = 15%, IC = 15%.

Discussion

All forms of dialytic intervention have their uses in the ICU population. The selection of the initial treatment modality is based on previous experience with specific patient groups. The patients with lower MAPs requiring pressor support and with increased A_2/A_1 ratios have continued to be those easiest and best served by C therapy. Since the needs of these critically ill patients frequently change from day to day, using a combination of therapy types has become a valuable option. This is reflected in the high percentage of therapy combinations used, not only within the C groups but also with the IC combinations. Figure 1 illustrates a single patient experience when exposed to multiple methods of support.

Ultimate mortality has not been shown to be affected by the choice of therapy. However, as has been reported by many authors, mortality in

Table 1. Average levels of blood urea nitrogen (BUN) and serum creatinine during therapy

Treatment	BUN, mg/dl	Creatinine, mg/dl
Continuous therapy	84.96 ± 21.97	4.19 ± 1.57
Intermittent/continuous therapy	94.50 ± 20.58	5.08 ± 1.35
Intermittent therapy	91.90 ± 24.97	5.56 ± 2.54

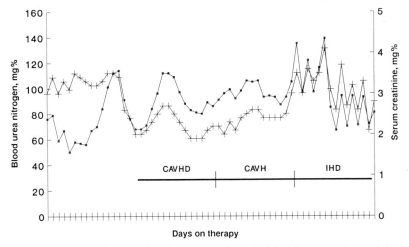

Fig. 1. Blood urea nitrogen (■) and serum creatinine (+) in a liver transplant recipient with acute renal failure, treated by a combination of renal replacement therapies.

those patients with acute renal failure is most affected by the patients' underlying disease and associated complications [2–6]. With three organ failures, Lohr's survival index predicts only a 19% chance of survival [4], which also parallels our experience. Using APACHE II, our patients group had scores in the 20–30 range (average = 26) and showed a survival of 32% last year. This is similar to Maher's description of a 21–26% survival of ICU patients with acute renal failure in the same APACHE II range [7].

Although no major impact has been made on survival of the patients reported in the present study, management of their complicated fluid, electrolyte and acid-base problems has been easier with C therapy. Based on our experience (n = 320 patients/3 years), the continued approach of treatment selection based on hemodynamic stability and high A_2/A_1 ratios is recommended.

References

1   Kraus W, Draper E, Wagner D, Zimmerman J: APACHE II: a severity of disease classification system. Crit Care Med 1985;13:818–829.
2   Beaman M, Turney J, Rodger R, McGonigle R, Adu D, Michael J: Changing pattern of acute renal failure. Q J Med 1989;269:857–866.
3   Cameron J: Acute renal failure – the continuing challenge. Q J Med 1986;228:337–343.
4   Corwin H, Bonventre J: Factors influencing survival in acute renal failure. Semin Dial 1989;2:220–225.
5   Gilium D, Dixon B, Yanover M, Kelleher S, Shapiro M, Benedetti R, Dillingham M, Paller M, Goldberg J, Tomford R, Gordon J, Conger J: The role of intensive dialysis in acute renal failure. Clin Nephrol 1985;25:249–254.
6   Lange H, Aeppli D, Bron D: Survival of patients with acute renal failure requiring dialysis after open heart surgery: Early prognostic indicators. Am Heart J 1987;113:1138–1143.
7   Maher E, Robinson K, Scoble J, Farrimond J, Browne D, Sweny P, Moorhead J: Prognosis of critically ill patients with acute renal failure: APACHE II score and other predictive factors. Q J Med 1989;269:857–866.

C. Bosworth, RN, Department of Hypertension and Nephrology,
The Cleveland Clinic Foundation, 9500 Euclid Ave., Cleveland,
OH 44195 (USA)

Sieberth HG, Mann H, Stummvoll HK (eds): Continuous Hemofiltration.
Contrib Nephrol. Basel, Karger, 1991, vol 93, pp 17–19

Outcome of Continuous Arteriovenous Hemofiltration in Acute Renal Failure

A Double-Center Comparative Study

Abdelmoniem A. Alarabi[a], *A. Brendolan*[b], *B.G. Danielson*[a],
F. Raimondi[b], *C. Ronco*[b], *B. Wikström*[a]

[a] Department of Internal Medicine, University Hospital, Uppsala, Sweden;
[b] Department of Nephrology, St. Bortolo Hospital, Vicenza, Italy

Continuous arteriovenous hemofiltration (CAVH) [1] is widely used as a treatment of choice for acute renal failure (ARF) in the critically ill intensive-care patients because it is simple and easy to perform even in infants [2]. CAVH allows the free administration of nutritional support [3, 4].

To evaluate the outcome of CAVH, this comparative retrospective study was carried out between the two centers of Uppsala, Sweden, and Vicenza, Italy.

Material and Methods

Fifty-six patients were included from each center during the period July 1987–July 1989. All patients were treated with CAVH in the postdilution mode (for the causes of their ARF, see table 1). Different types of hemofilters (polysulfone and polyacrylonitrile membranes) were used in each of the centers (table 2). Three types of vascular access were utilized in both centers, i.e. Buselmeier shunt (88% in Uppsala and 5% in Vicenza), femoral catheter (9% in Uppsala and 77% in Vicenza) and Scribner shunt (3% in Uppsala and 18% in Vicenza). Heparin (10–15 IU/kg body weight/h) was used as the standard anticoagulant in each center. The dose was adjusted by the partial thromboplastin time (PTT).

Results

The pretreatment serum urea (mean $\pm$ SD) level was significantly higher in the Uppsala patients ($p < 0.0001$; table 3). The duration of treatment was also significantly longer ($p < 0.05$) in the Uppsala patients. Heparin was administered in significantly larger doses ($p < 0.01$) in the Uppsala center; however, there were no significant differences between the daily mean systolic blood pressures or ultrafiltration volumes.

No complications were seen during CAVH treatment apart from filter clotting where in both centers the frequency of filter change was 0–4 in the individual patients during the total treatment duration (1–31 days).

Table 1. ARF causes and outcome of CAVH in two centers

ARF cause	Uppsala			Vicenza		
	patients	survival		patients	survival	
	n	n	%	n	n	%
Postsurgical	48	26	54	17	10	59
Postmedical	7	3	43	30	15	50
Major burns	1	1	100	2	1	50
Posttrauma	–	–	–	7	2	29
Total	56	30	54	56	28	50

Table 2. Types of filter (%) used for CAVH treatment

Membrane	Design	Uppsala	Vicenza
Polysulfone	Diafilter D10 (Amicon)	3	–
Polysulfone	Diafilter D20 (Amicon)	27	26
Polysulfone	Diafilter D30 (Amicon)	66	26
Polysulfone	Renaflo HF250 (Renal Systems)	5	–
Polyacrylonitrile	Biospal 1200S (Hospal)	–	31

Table 3. Comparison of the patients' data in the two centers

Parameter	Uppsala (n = 56)		Vicenza (n = 56)		p value
	mean ± SD	range	mean ± SD	range	
Age, years	58 ± 16	4.5 – 84	51 ± 15	17 – 81	<0.05
Serum urea, mmol/l	30 ± 14	4.5 – 92	18 ± 10	3 – 51	0.0001
BP, mm Hg	105 ± 16	40 – 140	107 ± 20	40 – 160	n.s.
PTT, s	51 ± 17	29 – 115	37 ± 10	0 – 81	0.001
Heparin, IU	675 ± 347	0 – 1,500	520 ± 237	0 – 1,200	<0.01
UF, l/24 h	14.3 ± 3	7.5 – 22.8	14 ± 5	3 – 29	n.s.
Treatment, days	8 ± 6	1 – 31	5 ± 5	0.75 – 21	<0.05
Age at death, years	61 ± 21	4.5 – 84	56 ± 13	17 – 81	n.s.

BP = Daily mean systolic blood pressure; UF = ultrafiltration; n.s. = nonsignificant.

The factors complicating ARF were almost similar in both centers where 30% of the patients were on mechanical respirator and 50% needed vasopressor drugs. However, in the Uppsala center, 23% of the patients were on aortic balloon pump. A total survival of 54 and 50% was obtained in Uppsala and Vicenza, respectively.

Discussion

When standard hemodialysis was used one third of high-risk ARF patients requiring intensive-care management survived and survival fell to one quarter in those requiring mechanical ventilation [5]. This might change if we consider the results from this study where a survival of 50–55% could be expected when CAVH was applied early as a treatment of choice for ARF in such critically ill intensive-care patients. This outcome is supported by previous studies [4, 6] with survivals of 45–55% using CAVH.

This study shows that the Uppsala patients were older (p < 0.05) and had a significantly higher pretreatment serum urea (p < 0.0001) than those in the Vicenza center. This suggests that the Uppsala patients were hyper-catabolic and more critically ill (e.g. 23% were on aortic balloon pump), requiring therefore a longer treatment duration. This fact may also indicate that treatment was initiated at an earlier stage in Vicenza patients. Although Uppsala patients had significantly higher PTT values (p < 0.001) than Vicenza patients, no bleeding complications were seen.

It is concluded from this study that a survival rate in the range of 50–55% can be expected when critically ill intensive-care patients with ARF are treated with CAVH. This indicates that CAVH is a valuable tool for treatment of ARF.

References

1   Kramer P, Wigger W, Rieger J, Matthaei D, Scheler F: Arteriovenous hemofiltration: A new and simple method for treatment of overhydrated patients resistant to diuretics. Klin Wochenschr 1977;55:1121–1122.

2   Ronco C: Continuous arteriovenous hemofiltration in infants; in Paganini EP (ed): Acute Continuous Renal Replacement Therapy. Boston, Nijhoff, 1986, chapt 12, pp 201–245.

3   Bartlett RH, Mault JR, Dechert RE, Palmer J, Swartz RD, Port FK: Continuous arteriovenous hemofiltration: Improved survival in surgical acute renal failure. Surgery 1986;100:400–408.

4   Weiss L, Danielson BG, Wikström B, Hedstrand U, Wahlberg J: Continuous arteri-ovenous hemofiltration in treatment of 100 critically ill patients with acute renal failure: Report on clinical outcome and nutritional aspects. Clin Nephrol 1989;31:184–189.

5   Wheeler DC, Feehaly J, Walls J: High risk acute renal failure. QJ Med 1986;61:977–984.

6   Alarabi AA, Danielson BG, Wikström B, Wahlberg J: Outcome of continuous arteri-ovenous hemofiltration (CAVH) in one centre. Ups J Med Sci 1989;94:299–303.

Dr. Abdelmoniem A. Alarabi, Department of Internal Medicine, University Hospital, S–751 85 Uppsala (Sweden)

Sieberth HG, Mann H, Stummvoll HK (eds): Continuous Hemofiltration.
Contrib Nephrol. Basel, Karger, 1991, vol 93, pp 20–22

Mortality in High-Risk Intensive-Care Patients with Acute Renal Failure Treated with Continuous Arteriovenous Hemofiltration

H.E. Sluiter, L. Froberg, J. van Dijl, J.G. Go

Department of Nephrology, University Hospital Groningen, The Netherlands

Acute renal failure in intensive-care patients carries a grim prognosis [1]. In catabolic patients with an unstable circulation, conventional intermittent hemodialysis (IHD) has met with only limited success.

The favorable experiences with the use of continuous renal replacement therapy in these critically ill patients in the early eighties [2, 3] led to the application of these techniques in the medical and surgical intensive-care facilities of the University Hospital of Groningen.

In this retrospective study, we wanted to evaluate mortality and causes of death in patients treated with continuous arteriovenous hemofiltration (CAVH) or slow continuous filtration (SCUF). Furthermore, the impact of several known risk factors for mortality was investigated.

Materials and Methods

Methods. Patient files were analyzed retrospectively from 110 consecutive intensive-care patients, treated with CAVH (SCUF) between October 1985 and July 1989. The following parameters were studied: previous illnesses, cause of renal failure, indication for intensive-care treatment, failure of other organ systems, details of CAVH technique, outcome, causes of death and complications of CAVH treatment.

Whenever possible, CAVH was performed using a standard technique. A Scribner shunt was used for vascular access. Using a 0.6-m^2 polyamide hollow-fiber filter (Gambro FH 66^R), an ultrafiltration rate of 600 ml/h was aimed at, to achieve a convective clearance of 10 ml/min. Sterile substitution fluid was administered in the postdilution mode. Anticoagulation was achieved by adding 600 U/h heparin. When necessary, a lower dose of heparin was given, or a predilution technique was employed. If sufficient clearance of solute could not be achieved with CAVH alone, bicarbonate IHD was performed, without fluid withdrawal.

Data are given as mean values (SEM). Possible differences between surviving and nonsurviving patient groups were analyzed with a χ^2 test.

Patients. Case records from 89 patients [56 men, 33 women, aged 62.7 (1.5) years] were included in the analysis. 30% of the patients were over 70 years of age. 57 patients had had major thoracic or abdominal surgery. Mechanical support of ventilation was needed in 91%, inotropic support in 80%. 83 patients had multiple (3 or more) organ failure. In the great majority the cause of acute renal failure was prerenal, in many cases complicated by the effects of nephrotoxic drugs or myoglobinuria, leading to acute tubular necrosis. Pretreatment plasma creatinine level was 510 (23) μmol/l, pretreatment urea, 37.5 (1.5) mmol/l.

Treatment was started with SCUF in 7 patients. 24 patients (27%) needed bicarbonate IHD after a period of CAVH. Median duration of CAVH was 8 days. Mean ultrafiltrate flow rate was 631 ml/h.

Results

50 patients (56.2%) died during the procedure or within 3 weeks after CAVH had been stopped. Prominent causes of death were cardiogenic shock (26%), sepsis (22%), malignancy (8%), liver failure (8%), intestinal bleeding and respiratory or neurological causes (6% each). In 18% of cases death was ascribed to multiple organ failure.

40 of 57 oliguric patients (diuresis < 300 ml/24 h) died, in contrast to 7 of 26 nonoliguric patients (p < 0.001). Of 18 patients with severe multiple organ failure 14 died, compared with 36 from the 71 patients with other indications (p < 0.05).

Comparing 39 surviving patients with the 50 (nonsurviving) patients, no single variable tested appeared to discriminate completely the patients from each other. No differences could be detected between patient groups with or without pretreatment creatinine > 500 μmol/l (n = 38), sepsis at start CAVH (n = 27), cardiac indication for CAVH (n = 13), history of severe trauma (n = 7), need for IHD (n = 24), previous history of renal insufficiency (n = 41), diabetes mellitus (n = 14), hypertension (n = 23), generalized arteriosclerosis (n = 27), myocardial infarction (n = 29), lung (n = 15) or liver disease (n = 27). There was no association for factors like age, plasma creatinine, urea, sodium or albumin, or for the number of organs failing at the start of treatment. The lack of a change in plasma urea levels after 3 days of CAVH likewise was not predictive of an adverse outcome.

Technique-related complications were coagulation of the extracorporeal circuit (in 44.3% of patients), bleeding (in 25.9%, mostly minor), and mineral and electrolyte disturbances (in 72.2%), of which hyponatremia (< 1330 mmol/l, in 30.1%), hypochloremia (< 95 mmol/l, in 44.4%) and hypocalcemia (< 2.10 mmol/l, in 31.7%) were the most frequent.

Discussion

In our patient population, treated with CAVH or SCUF, mortality was comparable with other reports, where similar [3, 4] or more intensive [1, 5, 6] continuous treatment modalities have been used. Death was not a direct consequence of renal failure. Very few data are available on the results of treatment with continuous versus intermittent renal replacement therapy. To avoid selection bias, and because in some patients additional IHD is necessary, a formal, prospective comparative study of CAVH and conventional daily, or alternate-day hemodialysis will be very difficult to perform, and will have to include several hundreds of carefully matched patients [1]. Likewise, it will be very difficult to demonstrate a possible superiority over CAVH in terms of patient survival of continuous forms of renal replacement therapies with higher clearance than CAVH, such as continuous arteriovenous hemodialysis or continuous pump-driven veno-venous hemofiltration/dialysis techniques. As was shown by the data presented, most patients in this study died, not as a consequence of renal failure, but from causes that could not be related to a state of uremia or overhydration.

In summary, we were able to confirm the negative impact on survival of a state of oliguria. In this retrospective study, no single variable tested appeared to be able to discriminate between survivors and nonsurvivors. Future studies, carried out prospectively, and analyzing longitudinal data, may provide more useful data to decide whether or not to start continuous renal replacement therapy in critically ill patients.

References

1 Simpson HKL, Allison MEM, Telfer ABM: Improving the prognosis in acute renal and respiratory failure. Renal Failure 1987;10:45–54.
2 Kramer P, Wigger W, Rieger J, Matthaei D, Scheler F: Arteriovenous hemofiltration: A new and simple method for treatment of overhydrated patients resistant to diuretics. Klin Wochenschr 1977;55:1121–1122.
3 Kaplan AA, Longnecker RE, Folkert VW: Continuous arteriovenous hemofiltration: A report of six month's experience. Ann Intern Med 1984;100:358–367.
4 Weiss L, Danielson BG, Wikstrom B, Hedstrand U, Wahlberg J: Continuous arteri-ovenous hemofiltration in the treatment of 100 critically ill patients with actue renal failure: Report on clinical outcome and nutritional aspects. Clin Nephrol 1989;31:184–189.
5 Wendon J, Smithies M, Sheppard M, Bullen K, Tinker J, Bihari D: Continuous high volume venous-venous haemofiltration in acute renal failure. Intensive Care Med 1989;15:358–363.
6 Stevens PE, Davies SP, Brown EA, Riley B, Gower PE, Kox W: Continuous arteri-ovenous haemodialysis in critically ill patients. Lancet 1988;ii:150–152.

Dr. H. E. Sluiter, Stichting Deventer Ziekenhuizen, Postbus 5001,
NL–7400 GC Deventer (The Netherlands)

Sieberth HG, Mann H, Stummvoll HK (eds): Continuous Hemofiltration.
Contrib Nephrol. Basel, Karger, 1991, vol 93, pp 23–28

Continuous Arteriovenous and Venovenous Hemodialysis in Critically Ill Patients

G.E. Schäfer, C. Döring, K. Sodemann, A. Russ, H.M. Schröder

Medizinische Klinik III, Städtische Kliniken, Offenbach, FRG

Intermittent hemodialysis may be detrimental in critically ill patients with acute renal failure (ARF) because hemodynamic instability frequently develops during conventional hemodialysis treatment (HD). Continuous arteriovenous hemofiltration (CAVH) was described by Kramer et al. [1] in 1977; the technique permits management of fluid and electrolyte balance even in hypotensive patients, but often is inefficient in the control of uremia in hypercatabolic states demanding the removal of large volumes of ultrafiltrate (20–30 liters/day).

Continuous hemodialysis (CHD), performed with arteriovenous (CAVHD) or pump-assisted venovenous (CVVHD) technique, is a recent modification of CAVH that combines ultrafiltration and dialysis. This alternative technique, proposed by Geronemus and Schneider [2] in 1984, provides efficient management of azotemia and control of fluid and electrolyte balance by diffusive and convective solute transport. To simplify an accurate control of dialysate flow we developed an automated fluid-balancing system for isovolumetric control of dialysate [3, 4]. The results and performance of this technique are illustrated in this preliminary clinical study.

Patients and Methods

Patients. CHD was performed in 62 patients with complicated ARF (36 men, 26 women, aged 24–86 years (mean 60.3 ± 14.3)). All patients had failure of 2, 3 or 4 organ systems and were considered to be poor candidates for conventional dialysis therapy. Fluid overload (53/62) was a common problem and contributed significantly to morbidity, associated with pulmonary edema (45/62) and vascular instability. Thirty-six patients required artificial ventilation and vasopressor infusions. Thirty-seven of the patients had a urine output of less than 400 ml/24 h.

Technical Data. CAVHD and CVVHD were performed on a continuous 24-hour basis for 1–38 days (mean duration of treatment 6.2 days/patient), using polyacrylonitrile hemofilters (Hospal, An-69 HF; 0.6 m²) and accompanying special blood tubing. In CHD an automated fluid balance system was established using double pump module BSM 22/VPM [4]. Isovolumetric balance of dialysate was realized by simultaneous application of two tubings

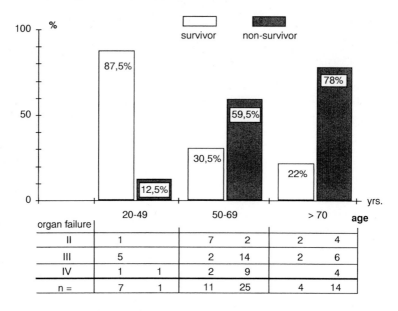

organ failure	20-49		50-69		>70	
II	1		7	2	2	4
III	5		2	14	2	6
IV	1	1	2	9		4
n =	7	1	11	25	4	14

Fig. 1. Outcome of ARF in 62 patients treated with CHD. Advancing age and number of coexistent organ failures are important risk factors.

inserted into the balancing pump. In CVVHD required fluid removal was controlled by an additional infusion pump. Vascular access was achieved by insertion of a Scribner shunt (4) or catheters inserted percutaneously with Seldinger wire technique via femoral artery (21) or jugular (20), subclavian (8) or femoral (9) vein.

Results

CHD was employed in 62 intensive-care patients with ARF. The total treatment time was 391 days (CAVHD 224 days (mean 9.7), CVVHD 167 days (mean 4.2) per patient). CAVHD and CVVHD were equally effective. The hourly filtrate loss ranged from 0 to 500 ml (mean 155 ± 141 ml).

Figure 1 gives details of the outcome in 62 patients with ARF and vascular instability. Twenty-two of the 62 patients survived (35.5%). The highest survival rate (87.5%) was found in the group of younger patients even in MOF, while the chance of survival declined with age and multiple organ systems failure. No death resulted from complications of CHD or as a direct result of ARF.

With dialysate flow rates of 1 liter/h and mean ultrafiltration of 2,940 ml/24 h all patients have reached consistent and controlled steady-state creatinine and urea levels despite hemodynamic instability, septicemia or surgery (fig. 2). CHD resulted in adequate control of uremia even in catabolic states and no patient required additional hemodialysis. At

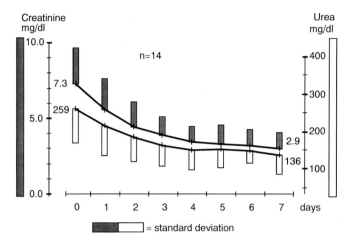

Fig. 2. Mean serum creatinine and urea levels during 7 days' CHD in 14 patients with ARF.

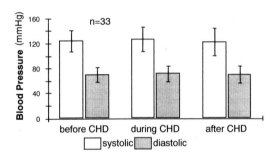

Fig. 3. Blood pressure in 33 patients with ARF and fluid overload during the first 24 h of CHD treatment; mean net fluid removal 3,735 ml.

dialysate flow rate of 15 ml/min the clearance of urea was 15.7 ml/min. It had never been necessary to increase the dialysate flow rate beyond 1 liter/h.

Particularly in critical patients CHD was tolerated without hemodynamic instability. In 33 extremely hypervolemic patients (fig. 3) blood pressure remained stable even at high ultrafiltration rates and a mean net fluid removal of 3,735 ml ($\pm 2,006$) was achieved during the first 24 h of treatment.

Figure 4 illustrates the maximum decline of blood pressure during the first 24 h of CHD in 33 patients with volume overload, correlated with the amount of fluid withdrawal. Even at a net loss of $> 5,000$ ml/24 h no critical drop in blood pressure was noted.

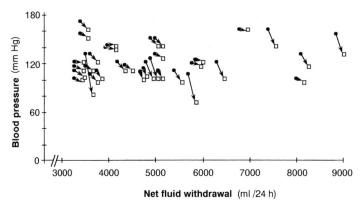

Fig. 4. Maximum decline of systolic blood pressure in ARF and fluid overload during the first 24 h of CHD (n = 33; mean net fluid removal 3,735 ml).

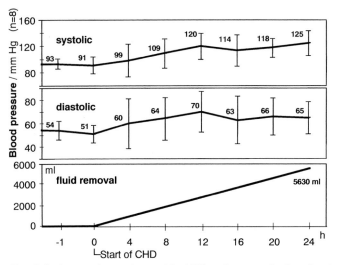

Fig. 5. In hypotensive patients with ARF, volume overload and pulmonary edema blood pressure rose significantly (p < 0.01) during CHD and a mean net fluid loss of 5,630 ml/24 h (n = 8).

To study the influence of CHD on hemodynamic stability, systolic and diastolic blood pressure before and during 24 h of treatment were recorded in 8 hypotensive patients with volume overload and pulmonary edema (fig. 5). During CHD a mean negative fluid balance of 5.6 liters was attained and systolic and diastolic blood pressure rose significantly (p < 0.01) while oxygen requirement decreased.

In all patients CHD allowed correction of electrolyte imbalance and adequate administration of energy and protein. The complication rate during CVVHD and CAVHD was low. Possibly due to heparinization, slight bleeding at the site of the vascular access was seen in 3 cases. Four times CHD had to be discontinued for overt bleeding from tracheostoma, pleural drainage or intestine. Heparin requirements were extremely variable (150–3,000 U/h, mean 1,080 ± 510 U/h).

Discussion

CAVHD or CVVHD provides efficient and flexible renal replacement therapy for critically ill patients. It is safe and reliable with less associated morbidity than other techniques. CHD assures an excellent tolerance to fluid removal and provides control of uremia and electrolyte balance: No patient required additional HD. In patients with ARF at dialysates flow rate of 1 liter/h a consistent and controlled steady-state creatinine and urea level is achieved within 3 days.

Because of intermittent hypotension most patients required support with dopamine and/or dobutamine before and during treatment. Particularly in critical patients CHD was tolerated without hemodynamic instability. Even in extremely hypervolemic states no critical drop in blood pressure was noted at a net fluid withdrawal of more than 5,000 ml during the first 24 h of treatment.

We consider CHD the treatment of choice for critically ill uremic patients at risk for cardiovascular instability, in fluid overload, respiratory failure, hypercatabolic state and electrolyte imbalance. The complication rate during CVVHD and CAVHD was low. No contraindications are known for CHD. Patients with bleeding risks must be monitored. Bedside supervision is necessary in excited patients and disturbance of consciousness.

The survival of 35.5% is remarkable in view of the severity of illness and declines with increasing age and the number of coexistent organ failures. In this extremely sick group of patients similar survival rates have been reported by others [5, 6]. Some favorable clinical results may be partly explained by the optimal tolerance to fluid removal, for water overload is common in patients with ARF and contributes significantly to mortality. CHD delivers a useful renal replacement therapy particularly in hypotensive and unstable patients.

After appropriate instruction, technique and control of CHD can be managed by the intensive-care nursing staff if closely supervised by a nephrologist. Although CHD may not alter the natural history of ARF complicating multiple organ failure, this modality reduces the morbidity associated with other forms of treatment and probably improves the chance of survival in some patients.

References

1   Kramer P, Wigger W, Rieger J, Matthaei D, Scheler F: Arteriovenous hemofiltration: A new simple method for treatment of overhydrated patients resistant to diuretics. Klin Wochenschr 1977;55:1121.

2   Geronemus R, Schneider N: Continuous arteriovenous hemodialysis: a new modality for treatment of acute renal failure. Trans Am Soc Artif Intern Organs 1984;30:610–613.

3   Sodemann K, Schäfer GE, Schröder H-M, Eckrich W, Schuh N, Förster H: Vorteile der bilanzierten kontinuierlichen arterio- bzw. veno-venösen Hämodialyse (CAVHD/CVVHD). Klin Wochenschr 1989;67(suppl 16):133–134.

4   Sodemann K, Niedenthal A, Russ A, Weber C, Schäfer GE: Automated fluid balance in continuous hemodialysis with blood safety module BSM 22/VPM; in Sieberth HG, Mann, H, Stummvoll HK (eds): Continuous Hemofiltration. Contrib Nephrol. Basel, Karger, 1991, vol 93, pp 184–192.

5   Schneider N, Geronemus R: Three-year study of continuous arteriovenous hemodialysis in acute renal failure (abstract). Xth Int Congr Nephrology, London, July 1987, p. 171.

6   Gibney RTN, Stollery DE, Lefebvre RE, Sharun CJ, Chan P: Continuous arteriovenous hemodialysis: an alternative therapy for acute renal failure associated with critical illness. Can Med Assoc J 1988;139:861–866.

Prof. Dr. med. G.E. Schäfer, Medizinische Klinik III, Städtische Kliniken,
Starkenburgring 66, D–W–6050 Offenbach am Main (FRG)

Sieberth HG, Mann H, Stummvoll HK (eds): Continuous Hemofiltration.
Contrib Nephrol. Basel, Karger, 1991, vol 93, pp 29–31

Survival in Patients Treated with Continuous Arteriovenous Hemodialysis for Acute Renal Failure and Chronic Renal Failure

Preliminary Observations

Robert P. Geronemus, Neil S. Schneider, Marguerite Epstein

Florida Medical Center, Lauderdale Lakes, Fla., USA

The diagnosis of acute renal failure (ARF) carries with it a very high mortality. This has remained so in spite of the advent of dialysis and other measures such as hyperalimentation [1, 2]. The continuous therapies (CAVH, CAVHD) have been touted as having advantages in the treatment of seriously ill patients with ARF or chronic renal failure (CRF) patients who are postoperative major surgery [3]. The advantages include superior cardiovascular stability, maintenance of fluid and electrolyte balance on a 24-hour basis, and the ability to deliver virtually unlimited quantitites of medications and hyperalimentation. While the continuous therapies certainly have the management of these patients much easier, it has been difficult to assess whether these advantages translate into improved survival.

We have managed renal failure patients since 1984 with CAVHD [4]. Our population consisted of an extremely elderly and sick sample. We are evaluating all patients who received CAVHD over the past 6 years using a simple clinical index of five complication factors. This index has previously been shown to be useful in assessing prognosis in ARF patients [1]. 110 patients have been analyzed to date and thus constitute the basis for preliminary conclusions.

Materials and Methods

The charts of all patients were retrospectively reviewed by one of us. Demographic data, diagnoses, and outcome were recorded. Presence or absence of five complicating factors (hypotension, assisted ventilation, gastrointestinal dysfunction, congestive heart failure, proven or suspected sepsis) were recorded as of the time of initiation of dialysis.

Patients were treated with CAVHD using previously published techniques. Most patients were treated with the 0.5 m² flat plate AN-69S dialyzer (Hospal Medical Corp.). Access was general via femoral arterial and venous cannulae with 7 French inside diameter × 4.5 inch length (MedComp, Harleysville, Pa).

Table 1. Distribution of patients per category

Number of factors present	Number of patients		
	total	ARF	CRF
0	4	1	3
1	10	10	0
2	21	17	4
3	37	31	6
4	29	27	2
5	9	9	0

Table 2. Survival statistics

Number of factors present	Percent survival		
	total	ARF	CRF
0	75	100	65
1	60	60	—
2	43	41	50
3	30	26	50
4	7	7	0
5	11	11	—

Results

Of the 110 patients evaluated to date, 82 were male and 28 female. Mean age was 73 years (range 39–90). The distribution of patients per category is shown in table 1. Sixty-eight percent of the patients had 3–5 complication factors with the average number of factors per patient being 3.4; the sample itself consisted of mostly seriously ill patients. There were 95 patients with ARF and 15 with CRF. Overall survival was 29%, survival in the ARF patients was 26%. Table 2 shows survival statistics for all patients, ARF patients, and CRF patients as a function of the number of complication factors.

Conclusions

Survival was inversely related to the number of complication factors present, although there was little difference in survival in the sickest patients with 4–5 factors. When compared to the previously published data by Lohr et al. [1], the overall survival was similar (29% in our study versus 25% in Lohr's study). However, the age of our patients was more than 15 years older and our patients were sicker, having on average 3.4

complication factors versus 2.6 in the previous study. These data suggest that renal failure patients treated with CAVHD have improved survival over those treated with traditional methods.

References

1   Lohr JW, McFarlane MJ, Grantham JJ: Clinical index to predict survival in acute renal failure patients requiring dialysis. Am J Kidney Dis 1988;11:254–59.
2   Eliahou HE, Bartlet RH, Schrier RW, et al: Acute renal failure revisited. The full circle in ARF mortality. Trans Am Soc Artif Intern Organs 1984;30:700–703.
3   Lauer A, Saccaggi C, Ronco C, et al: Continuous arteriovenous hemofiltration in the critically ill patient. Ann Intern Med 1983;99:455.
4   Geronemus R, Schneider N: Continuous arteriovenous hemodialysis: A new modality for treatment of acute renal failure. Trans Am Soc Artif Intern Organs 1984;30:610–613.

Robert P. Geronemus, MD, Florida Medical Center, 4900 West Oakland Park Boulevard, Suite 302, Lauderdale Lakes, FL 33313 (USA)

Sieberth HG, Mann H, Stummvoll HK (eds): Continuous Hemofiltration.
Contrib Nephrol. Basel, Karger, 1991, vol 93, pp 32–38

Acute Renal Failure Associated with Multiple Organ Failure: Pump-Assisted Continuous Venovenous Hemofiltration, the Ultimate Treatment Modality

B. Canaud[a], *J.P. Cristol*[a], *C. Berthelemy*[a], *K. Klouche*[b], *J.J. Beraud*[b], *C. Mion*[a]

[a]Nephrology Intensive Care Unit, and [b]Metabolic Intensive Care Unit,
Lapeyronie University Hospital, Montpellier, France

Acute renal failure (ARF), a common feature of multiple organ failure (MOF), is usually associated with two or more life-threatening complications (hypotension or shock, liver failure, sepsis, respiratory distress, coagulopathy). Treatment of ARF in this context is hazardous, indeed impossible with conventional methods. Slow continuous renal replacement therapy (CRRT) preventing rapid fluid and/or solute removal is therefore mandatory [1–4]. Continuous arteriovenous hemofiltration (CAVH) popularized by Kramer has proved very useful in the management of these precarious patients [5–7]. CAVH, however, may be hampered in MOF patients by two facts: a hypercatabolic state, a basic feature in this context, which produced large amount of urea exceeding CAVH removal capacity; the limitation of ultrafiltration rate and urea clearances to 10–12 liters/24 h due to the low spontaneous flow regimen [7, 8]. To overcome these shortcomings, yet in keeping with the concept of continuous therapy, several solutions have been proposed: optimal blood circuit and filter design increasing filtration rate, suction-assisted CAVH, combined with low flow dialysate in CAVHD or CAVHDF [9–11]. Finally, pump-driven venovenous system or combined therapy (CAVH plus intermittent HD) have been proposed as a more versatile alternative [12, 13].

Basic urea kinetic concepts applied to CRRT allow us to easily predict the 'dialysis dose' (daily integrated clearance) needed to maintain urea level within a suitable range (20–25 mmol/l) at any degree of urea generation rate. For example, the daily integrated clearance required to maintain the urea level at around 20 mmol/l for a patient producing 300–600 μmol/min of urea should be 15–30 ml/min (20–40 liters/day). According to this basic concept, we surmised that the pump-assisted continuous venovenous hemofiltration system (CVVH) would offer a more versatile and adequate method to optimize individual fluid volume exchange.

This study reports on our experience of using CVVH as a specific treatment modality of ARF in MOF patients.

Material and Methods

Patients. 32 patients (15 males, 17 females, age 57.3 ± 15.7 years) referred to us for ARF with associated MOF (ARF plus at least 2 other system failures: severe hypotension, shock, liver, respiratory, sepsis) were included in this treatment study protocol.

ARF Etiology. Anuric ARF developed secondary to abdominal surgery in 18 patients, sepsis episodes 19, vascular surgery 16, cardiogenic shock 3, traumatic rhabdomyolysis 3, liver failure 3. Several causes may have been associated in the same patient. Severe acute tubular necrosis was the most common finding in biopsied patients.

ARF and MOF. Vital system or organ failure associated with ARF were as follows: respiratory failure requiring mechanical ventilatory assistance in 27 (82%); cardiocirculatory shock requiring inotropic and/or vasoacting drugs in 26 (81%); extracellular fluid overload (> 10% of body weight) in 23 (72%); severe uncontrolled sepsis in 20 (63%); liver failure with jaundice in 11 (34%); hemorragic or coagulopathy syndrome in 4 (13%). Simplified acuity score (SAS) at time of ICU admission was 16.5 for the whole population.

CVVH Technique. CVVH was initiated usually on ICU admission when ARF with associated MOF was confirmed and interrupted either when the patient's clinical condition improved permitting his transfer to conventional bicarbonate dialysis or due to the patient's death. CVVH was performed via a venovenous circuit using a double-head-pump monitoring module (BSM22, Hospal, Basel, Switzerland) to secure extracorporeal circuit and fluid volume balance as shown in figure 1 [12, 13]. The blood pump maintained a constant blood flow rate at 100–200 ml/min. The infusate pump was used to compensate for the ultrafiltration and the body weight loss. Actual and cumulative infusate flow were displayed on the BSM22. Bicarbonate infusate was batch prepared on-site as already described in 30 liter closed plastic bags held in a rigid container [14]. A 0.22-μm disk filter was inserted on the infusion line just before the injection site of the substitution fluid in the venous bubble trap. Ultrafiltration flow rate was adjusted by means of blood flow rate and venous return pressure to maintain prescription order. Highly permeable hemofilters (Biospal 2400s, AN69 plate membrane; Filtral 12, AN69, capillary filter) were used ad libitum until filtration rate reached an unacceptably low value or clotting occurred. Daily fluid volume exchanged (15–40 liters/24 h) was tailored to the individual patients needs according to urea generation rate in order to maintain blood urea concentration at around 20 mmol/l. Net daily fluid removal obtained from the ultrafiltration/infusate fluid volume imbalance was defined according to extracellular fluid volume status. Standard heparin or low-molecular-weight heparin were used to prevent clotting of filter and blood lines in 20 and 9 patients, respectively. Three patients with hepatic failure had received no antithrombotic agent. Vascular access was obtained from percutaneous catheterization of deep vein: femoral 19 (59%), internal jugular vein 12 (39%), subclavian 1 (3%). Total parenteral nutrition was performed in all patients.

Patient Follow-Up. Simplified acuity score (SAS) derived from acute physiology score (APS) was determined at the time of ICU admission [15]. Vital signs (blood pressure, heart rate, temperature, breath rate) were recorded hourly on the patient's logchart. Body weight

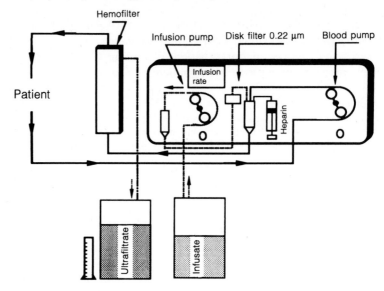

Fig. 1. CVVH apparatus set-up consisting of a double-head-pump monitor (BSM 22, Hospal) with safety alarms: one is a blood pump monitoring module, the other is an infusate pump monitoring module (0.1–2.0 liters/h). Ultrafiltrate is collected in a 30-liter plastic container. Bicarbonate infusate produced on-site stored in a 30-liter closed plastic bag hold in a rigid container. A disk filter is interposed on the infusion line.

was recorded hourly with an electronic bed scale. Ultrafiltration rate collected in a graduated cylinder was measured every hour. Infusion rate was calculated from infusate tank weight changes every hour. Fluid volume balance was established hourly from ultrafiltration and infusion volume. Infusate flow was therefore adapted hourly to follow exchange volume prescription. Daily usual chemistry (urea, creatinine, Na, K, Cl, HCO_3, Ca, PO_4) was obtained from blood and ultrafiltrate. Hematology and clotting parameters were obtained daily.

Calculations and Statistics. SAS was calculated from a scoring scale ($-4, 0, +4$) applied to a set of clinical and chemical selected criteria [15]. Simplified urea kinetic monitoring was done using the total amount of ultrafiltrate collected daily and blood urea changes. Values were expressed as mean values $\pm$ SE. Wilcoxons signed-rank test was used to compare mean group of values. $p < 0.05$ was used as level of significance.

Results

Cumulative time spent on CVVH was 169 days (1–21 days) yielding to 5.3 days/patient. 73 filters were used during this period giving a life span of 2.3 days/filter. The overall survival rate computed by the life-table analysis method is presented in figure 2. The risk of dying was maximum within the first 10 days, thereafter survival plateaued at around 20%.

SAS value was 16.5 ± 0.8 for the whole group of patients. It was significantly higher for dying than for surviving patients (17.5 ± 0.7 vs.

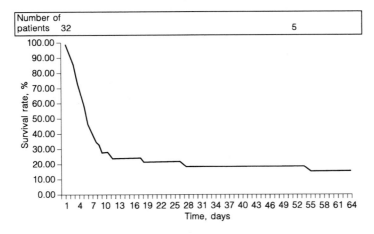

Fig. 2. Survival rate according to life table analysis in 32 patients with ARF associated with MOF treated by CVVH. Risk of dying is maximum within the first 10 days and thereafter survival rate plateaus at around 20%.

11.2 ± 2.4). The ultrafiltration volume necessary to maintain blood urea levels at around 20 mmol/l was 23.3 ± 4.1 liters/24 h ranging from 15 to 42 liters/24 h with an infusate volume of 21.5 ± 3.6 liters/24 h. Urea generation rate decreased from 400 to 250 μmol/min and protein catabolic rate from 2.4 to 1.25 g/kg/day after the 10th day of CVVH (fig. 3). Total parenteral nutrition consisted of a caloric intake of 35 ± 10 kcal/kg/day with a nitrogen intake of 11 ± 3 g/day. Blood urea concentrations decreased from 40 to 20 and blood creatinine from 600 to 250 at the steady state reached after 4 days of CVVH. Serum potassium was stabilized at around 3.75 mmol/l. Metabolic acidosis was easily corrected, bicarbonate concentration steadily increased from 21 to 27 mmol/l after 8 days. Sodium concentration was normalised and remained at around 137 mmol/l. Fluid volume overload noted in 25/32 patients at initiation of CVVH was corrected in all patients with a net negative fluid volume removal of 7.5 kg. Hemoglobin concentration, leukocytes and platelet counts did not change significantly during the course of the disease, averaging 9.5 g/dl, 20 and $150 \times 10^3/\text{mm}^3$, respectively. Sytemic blood pressure was maintained in the range of 100/55 mm Hg, in spite of hemodynamic instability and constant fluid removal (fig. 4). The use of inotropic and/or vasoacting drugs required in 26/32 patients was usually reduced after the 4th or 5th days.

Discussion

ARF with MOF raises the crucial question of whether to treat such poor prognosis and high-risk patients [4]. Initiating treatment of ARF in

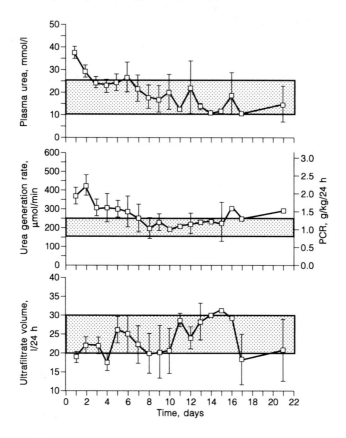

Fig. 3. Plasma urea level (upper branch), urea generation rate (μmol/min) and protein catabolic rate (g/kg/24 h) (middle panel) and daily ultrafiltration volume (liters/24 h) as function of time. As shown, plasma urea concentration was maintained at the optimal level in spite of high protein catabolism with daily fluid volume exchange of around 23–25 liters.

this context is very hazardous, and conventional intermittent dialysis would be challenging if not impossible because of cardiovascular instability. Continuous low flow renal replacement therapies (CAVH, CAVHD, CVVH, CVVHD) are recognized as the best alternative treatment in these patients [1, 2, 5, 7, 11]. In keeping with this key concept of slow continuous therapy, CVVH offers a more versatile method which permits tailoring the 'dose therapy' to the patient's actual needs. On-site batch preparation of bicarbonate substitution fluid virtually suppresses any limitation in fluid volume prescription. Mean daily fluid volume exchanged was 22.3 liters but had to be increased up to 42 liters in highly catabolic patients: such a high

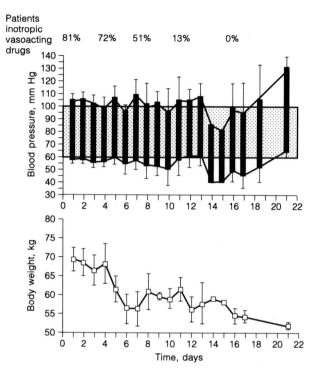

Fig. 4. Blood pressure (upper panel) and body weight changes expressed as daily mean value according to time. Inotropic and vasoactive drug use was reduced after 6 days.

exchange volume could certainly not be obtained with arteriovenous methods. Bicarbonate buffered infusate instead of lactate responds better to the metabolic requirements and cardiovascular instability of MOF patients. Fluid volume handling was simplified by the use of 30-liter plastic bags changed once or twice a day.

CVVH, the ultimate treatment possibility for ARF with associated MOF was successfully performed in this group of high-risk patients. Despite a poor outcome, the 20% life survival rate compared favorably with published series and can be accepted as a positive result in this group of desperately ill patients.

Efficacy of CVVH, a direct function of daily fluid volume exchange, was achieved even in hypercatabolic patients (urea generation rate averaging 400 μmol/min) with the ultrafiltration volume reaching 40 liters/day. Continuous renal replacement therapy facilitated parenteral nutrition by allowing adequate caloric and nitrogen intake in the absence of fluid restriction. Satisfactory correction of acidosis and plasma electrolyte concentration was obtained. Cardiovascular stability was maintained in an acceptable range with a reduction of inotropic and vasoacting drugs.

In conclusion, despite its apparent technical complexity, CVVH was easily implemented in our intensive care unit and integrated with benefit in the complex care of ARF with associated MOF.

References

1   Olbricht C, Mueller C, Schurek HJ, Stolte H: Treatment of acute renal failure in patients with multiple organ failure by continuous spontaneous hemofiltration. Trans ASAIO 1982;28:33.
2   Bartlett RH, Mault JR, Dechert RE, Palmer J, Swartz RD, Port FK: Continuous arteriovenous hemofiltration: Improved survival in surgical acute renal failure? Surgery 1986;100:400–408.
3   Sigler MH, Teehan BP, Van Valkenburgh D: Solute transport in continuous hemodialysis: A new treatment for acute renal failure. Kidney Int 1987;32:562–571.
4   Paganini EP: Continuous renal replacement therapy in acute renal failure. Is it prolonging the inevitable or changing the outcome? Nephrol News Issues 1989;19.
5   Kramer P, Bohler J, Kehr A, Grone HJ, Schraeder J, Matthaie O, Scheler F: Intensive care potential of continuous arteriovenous hemofiltration. Trans ASAIO 1982;28:28–32.
6   Geronemus R, Schneider N: Continuous arteriovenous hemodialysis: A new modality for treatment of acute renal failure. Trans ASAIO 1984;30:610–612.
7   Lauer A, Saccaggi A, Ronco C, Belledonne M, Glabman S, Bosch J: Continuous arteriovenous hemofiltration in the critically ill patient. Ann Intern Med 1983;99:455–460.
8   Golper TA, Ronco C, Kaplan AA: Continuous arteriovenous hemofiltration: Improvements, modifications, and future directions. Semin Dial 1988;1:50.
9   Kaplan AA, Longnecker RE, Folker VW: Suction-assisted continuous arteriovenous hemofiltration. Trans ASAIO 1983;29:408–412.
10 Kaplan AA: Predilution vs. postdilution for continuous arteriovenous hemofiltration. Trans ASAIO 1985;31:28–31.
11 Ronco C, Brendolan A, Bragantini L, Chiaramonte S, Dell'Aquila R, Fabris A, Feriani M, Milan M, La Greca G: Arteriovenous hemodiafiltration associated with continuous arteriovenous hemofiltration: A combined therapy for acute renal failure in the hypercatabolic patients; in La Greca G, Fabris A, Ronco C (eds): CAVH. Proc Int Symp CAVH. Milano, Wichtig Editore, 1986, pp 171–183.
12 Canaud B, Beraud JJ, Mion C: Pump assisted continuous veno-venous hemofiltration (PACVVH): A more flexible mode of acute uremia treatment in severely ill patients; in La Greca G, Fabris A, Ronco C (eds): CAVH. Proc Int Symp CAVH. Milano, Wichtig Editore, 1986, pp 185–189.
13 Canaud B, Garred LJ, Cristol JP, Aubas S, Béraud JJ, Mion C: Pump assisted continuous venovenous hemofiltration for treating acute uremia. Kidney Int 1988;S24:154–156.
14 Mion C, Canaud B: 'On-site' preparation of sterile apyrogenic electrolyte solutions for hemofiltration and hemodiafiltration; in Cambi V (ed): Short Dialysis. Boston, Nijhoff, 1987; vol 12, pp 261–291.
15 Knaus WA, Wagner DP, Loirat P, Zimmerman JE: A comparison of intensive care in the USA and France. Lancet 1982;ii:642–646.

Dr. Bernard Canaud, Division of Nephrology, Intensive Care Unit,
Lapeyronie University Hospital, F–34059 Montpellier (France)

Sieberth HG, Mann H, Stummvoll HK (eds.): Continuous Hemofiltration.
Contrib Nephrol. Basel, Karger, 1991, vol 93, pp 39–41

Nitrogen Balance in Postsurgical Patients with Acute Renal Failure on Continuous Arteriovenous Hemofiltration and Total Parenteral Nutrition[1]

Cinda S. Chima[a], *Lisa Meyer*[a], *Robert Heyka*[a], *Cindy Bosworth*[a],
A. Christine Hummel[a], *A. Werynski*[b], *Emil Paganini*[a], *P. Verdi*[a]

[a]The Cleveland Clinic Foundation Cleveland, Ohio, USA; [b]Institute of Biocybernetics
and Biomedical Engineering, Polish Academy of Sciences, Warsaw, Poland

Acute renal failure (ARF) in the postsurgical patient commonly occurs subsequent to multiple organ system failure secondary to sepsis or an ischemic event. CAVH therapy permits the provision of nutritional support in these unstable patients. While Bartlett and co-workers have examined energy needs using indirect calorimetry, limited information exists regarding the protein needs of these patients.

This study was undertaken to: (a) estimate energy and protein needs of post surgical patients in ARF on CAVH and TPN using standard equations for nutrition assessment of critically ill patients; (b) determine urea nitrogen appearance (UNA), total nitrogen appearance (TNA) and protein catabolic rate (PCR) through direct measurement of body losses and body pool nitrogen changes; (c) compare estimated and actual PCR, and (d) determine the correlation between UNA and TNA.

Methods

Sixteen postoperative subjects in ARF on CAVH and TPN were studied (8 males, 8 females, mean age 65 years, mean APACHE score of 21), nonsurgical patients, patients on enteral or oral feedings, those receiving other forms of dialysis therapy, or with chest tubes or major blood losses were excluded.

CAVH access was via cannulation of the femoral artery and vein. Rates were controlled via IVAC pump with mean ultrafiltration rate of 15,393 ± 5,329 ml/day or 640 ml/h. Replacement was via venous (post ultrafiltration) port using a standardized ultrafiltration fluid. There was no interruption of CAVH during any study period.

[1] Bibliography available from the author by request.

Table 1. Estimated needs, actual intake, and measured PCR in CAVH patients

	Protein g	Nitrogen g	kcal	kcal/N
Estimated needs	105 ± 20	16.7 ± 3.2	2,548 ± 498	153:1
per kg	1.5 ± 0.25	0.24 ± 0.04	37 ± 6	
Actual TPN	97 ± 32	15.5 ± 5.1	2,588 ± 564	167:1
per kg	1.4 ± 0.5	0.22 ± 0.1	36 ± 6	
PCR-TNA	120.5 ± 45	19.3 ± 7.2	–	–
per kg	1.8 ± 0.75	0.29 ± 0.12	–	–

Energy and protein needs were estimated using the Harris-Benedict and Long (150 kcal/ g N) equations, respectively. Parenteral nutrition support was adjusted to provide estimated energy and protein needs.

Ultrafiltrate, nasogastric tube losses, and urine (if any) was collected for each 24-hour study period and aliquots were analyzed for urea (urease method) creatinine (Jaffe method) and uric acid (uricase method). None of the subjects passed stool during the study periods. Pool volume and change in body urea and nonurea nitrogen (uric acid, creatinine) were also determined. Change in body pool nitrogen was determined as:

Delta $M = Vpost \cdot Cpost - Vpre \cdot Cpre$,

where M is solute (urea, uric acid, creatinine) body pool change over 24 h, and Vpost and Cpost are the postcollection distribution volume and blood plasma concentration, respectively.

TNA over 24 hours was calculated as:

$TNA = UN + CN + AN + delta\ M.$

UNA over 24 h was calculated as:

$UNA = UN + delta\ MUN,$

where MUN is the urea nitrogen body pool change over 24 h.

Data were analyzed and Pearson correlation coefficients determined using the SAS System, SAS Institute, Cary, N.C.

Results

A total of thirty 24-hour collections were conducted on the 16 subjects (table 1). TNA and UNA were strongly correlated ($r = 0.99$, $p < 0.001$). Mean NB was $-3.5 ± 7.9$ g; 14 patients were in negative NB. PCR was significantly, though not strongly correlated with estimated protein needs ($r = 0.50$, $p < 0.008$).

Discussion

A number of mathematical models have been developed to evaluate the effects of hemodialysis and enhance the management of the patient with renal failure. Because of differences in dialyzer clearances and impact of dialysis on urea generation, it is not clear that equations used to describe the relationship between TNA and UNA in hemodialysis patients are applicable to CAVH.

It has been suggested that CAVH is an appropriate dialysis therapy for use in primary and secondary health care institutions due to its simplicity and the fact that it requires little specialized equipment. In this study we attempted to replicate nutritional assessment techniques used in such hospitals (Harris-Benedict and Long's equations) and compare them to direct quantification of nitrogen appearance. Although PCR for the group was underestimated using assessment calculations, PCR was underestimated in some individuals and overestimated in others.

One disadvantage in this study was that the study periods were relatively brief (1–5 days, mode = 2 days) and daily PCR highly variable. It may be that standard nutrition assessment techniques would be better predictors of mean PCR measured over longer time periods.

Conclusion

We conclude that UNA and TNA are highly correlated in patients on CAVH. Standard assessment techniques may be successful in predicting mean protein needs in groups, but in this study did not correlate well with daily PCR in individuals. Studies of longer duration are needed to evaluate the clinical significance of these differences, and daily variation of PCR in patients on CAVH.

Cinda S. Chima, RD, Nutrition Services, Metrohealth Medical Center, 3395 Scranton Road, Cleveland, OH 44109 (USA)

Sieberth HG, Mann H, Stummvoll HK (eds): Continuous Hemofiltration.
Contrib Nephrol. Basel, Karger, 1991, vol 93, pp 42–46

Continuous Hemofiltration and Hemodiafiltration in the Management of Multiple Organ Failure

Hiroyuki Hirasawa, Takao Sugai, Yoshio Ohtake, Shigeto Oda,
Hidetoshi Shiga, Kenichi Matsuda, Nobuya Kitamura

Department of Emergency and Critical Care Medicine, Chiba University School of
Medicine, Chiba, Japan

Multiple organ failure (MOF) remains a serious problem in modern medical practice. In the management of MOF, various blood purifications such as hemodialysis (HD), peritoneal dialysis (PD) and hemoadsorption (HA) are essential [1, 2]. Continuous hemofiltration (CHF) has been widely applied in the management of critically ill patients [3, 4]. Recently, it has been reported that not only CHF but also continuous hemodiafiltration (CHDF) are effective in the treatment of acute renal failure (ARF) [5]. The present study was undertaken to evaluate the efficacy of CHF and CHDF in the management of critically ill patients, especially in the management of MOF.

Subjects and Methods

Forty-three patients with MOF, ARF and acute impairment of chronic renal failure who were treated with CHF and/or CHDF for at least 48 h during the period from October, 1985 and July, 1990, entered the study. CHF and/or CHDF were performed as follows. For the blood access, an intravenous double lumen catheter was inserted if the patient's body weight was above 25 kg, and the indwelling catheters were inserted to an artery and a vein if the body weight was less than 25 kg. A hemofilter HF-0.3U or 0.6U with the membrane area of 0.3 and 0.6 m^2, respectively (Toray, Japan), was used. A special bedside console for CHF and CHDF with a blood pump, a filtration controller, a syringe pump for anticoagulant and various monitoring systems (Hemoflex, Ube Company, Japan) was used. A protease inhibitor, nafamostat mesilate or low-molecular-weight heparin or heparin was administered as anticoagulant in the dose of 0.1 mg/kg/h, 2.5 U/kg/h and 2–4 U/kg/h, respectively [4]. Filtration rate was approximately 100 ml/kg/day. Mixture of 50% glucose and amino acid solution for total parenteral nutrition, electrolyte solution as well as fresh frozen plasma were administered as replacement fluid in the way of postdilution. In the case of CHDF sterile bicarbonate dialysate was used with the flow rate of 500 ml/h. Therefore, the filtration controller for a patient with the body weight of 50 kg was set to be approximately 700 ml/h (200 ml of filtrate plus 500 ml of dialysate).

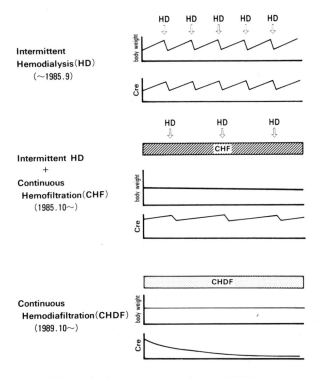

Fig. 1. Changes in the management of anuric MOF patients.

The survival of the patients, the efficacy of CHF and/or CHDF, bleeding complication during CHF and/or CHDF with anticoagulants were studied. Since our previous report [4] indicated that better nutritional support for anuric MOF patients could be obtained with the simultaneous application of CHF to remove excess‐water given as carrier of TPN, we investigated the sufficiency rate of energy intake (energy intake with total parenteral nutrition/ energy expenditure measured with the indirect calorimetry) [6]. Also studied were the sieving coefficients of various causative humoral mediators of MOF including complement component C_{3a}, thromboxane B_2, granulocyte elastase, lipid peroxide and tumor necrosis factor (TNF).

Results

There were 18 surgical and 17 medical MOF patients treated with CHF and/or CHDF during the study period, of whom 9 (50%) and 9 (53%) survived, respectively. All of 6 ARF patients and 2 patients with acute impairment of chronic renal failure survived. As shown in figure 1, we first applied CHF for the management of water and electrolyte among anuric MOF. However, intermittent HD was mandatory to remove metabolic waste products and was performed 2–3 times a week. However, most critically ill patients could not tolerate HD even though no water was removed during HD. On the other hand, we could avoid intermittent HD for the removal of waste products when we performed CHDF, which had been applied to critically ill MOF patients since October, 1989. CHDF could maintain water and electrolytes balance and remove metabolic waste products without intermittent HD. Thus, even most critically ill patients could be treated with CHDF alone. The incidence of bleeding complications caused by the prolonged administration of anticoagulant was 4% (1/23) with nafamostate mesilate, 29% (5/17) with low-molecular-weight heparin, and 67% (8/12) with heparin. Those data indicate that nafamostate mesilate is the anticoagulant of the choice for CHF and CHDF on critically ill patients.

The sufficiency rate of energy intake was $73.3 \pm 14.7\%$ with TPN alone and $102.1 \pm 8.1\%$ with TPN and simultaneous CHF and CHDF ($p < 0.01$), indicating that better nutritional management can be performed with TPN and simultaneous CHF and CHDF. The sieving coefficients of C_{3a}, thromboxane B_2, granulocyte elastase, lipid peroxide and TNF during CHF were 77.5, 50.5, 2.1, 42.2 and 52.2%, respectively, indicating that those humoral mediators except granulocyte elastase could be effectively removed with CHF.

Discussion

CHF has been applied in the treatment of MOF patients and has been found to be very effective in the management of water and electrolyte metabolism and in the nutritional management in anuric MOF [4]. However, we noticed that CHF was not satisfactory to remove metabolic waste products and that intermittent HD was mandatory to remove them [4]. It may be possible to remove even metabolic waste products with CHF if huge amount of filtrate was obtained. However, Davenport [7] recently reported that CHF with large volume of filtrate had an adverse effect of the loss of important molecules such as carnitine to cause serious complications. Furthermore, Davenport and Roberts [8] also reported that amino acid given as nutrient could be lost into filtrate during CHF and that this loss of amino acid was proportional to the amount of filtrate. These results indicate that CHF with large volumes of filtrate is not recommended in the management of MOF.

CHDF has the advantage of CHF and in addition can remove the waste products effectively. Therefore, if a patient with MOF is anuric and his BUN and serum creatinine level is not so high (BUN is less than 100 mg/dl and serum creatinine is less than 7 mg/dl), CHF sould be applied. If an anuric MOF patient shows high BUN and high serum creatinine level, CHDF should be chosen in place of CHF.

Basically, our method is a continuous venovenous hemofiltration (CVVH). Some investigators prefer continuous arteriovenous hemofiltration (CAVH) to CVVH because of its simplicity in that it does not need a blood pump [5, 9]. However, our previous experience [4] indicated that CVVH can be more applicable even to the critically ill patient. Bleeding complication is one of the serious complications during CHF and CHDF [9]. Our results clearly indicate that we can avoid the bleeding complication during CHF and CHDF when we use the protease inhibitor, nafamostat mesilate, and that, therefore, nafamostate mesilate is suitable for the anticoagulant during CHF and CHDF.

Humoral mediators draw much attention as the causative substances of MOF. The results of our study suggest that many causative humoral mediators could be effectively removed with CHF and that, therefore, CHF and CHDF might be beneficial in this respect in the management of MOF.

In conclusion, CHF and CHDF are safe and effective blood purifications in the management of MOF. The efficiacy of CHF and CHDF in the management of MOF can be summarized as follows: (1) maintenance of water and electrolyte balance; (2) removal of metabolic waste products; (3) removal of causative substances of MOF such as humoral mediators. CHDF is superior to CHF in terms of the removal of metabolic waste products and intermittent HD can be avoided with CHDF. Therefore, CHDF is the blood purification of first choice in the management of the most critically ill MOF patient who shows high BUN and serum creatinine levels.

References

1   Hirasawa H, Odaka M, Kobayashi H, Soeda K, Kobayashi S, Murotani N, Ito Y, Isono K: Hemopurification in the treatment of multiple organ failure; in Nose Y, Kjellstrand C, Ivannovich P (eds): Progress in Artificial Organs – 1985. Cleveland, ISAO Press, 1986, pp 730–734.
2   Hirasawa H, Odaka M, Sugai T, Ohtake Y, Inaba H, Tabata Y, Kobayashi H, Isono K: Prognostic value of serum osmolality gap in patients with multiple organ failure treated with hemopurification. Artif Organs 1988;12:382–387.
3   Barzilay E, Kessler D, Lesmes C, Lev A, Weksler N, Berlot G: Sequential plasmafilter-dialysis with slow continuous hemofiltration: Additional treatment for sepsis-induced AOSF patients. J Crit Care 1988;3:163–166.
4   Hirasawa H, Sugai T, Ohtake Y, Oda S, Shiga H, Odaka M: Continuous hemofiltration (CHF) in the treatment of anuric multiple organ failure (MOF). Artif Organs 1990;14 (suppl 2):117–119.
5   van Geelen JA, Vincent HH, Schalekamp MADH: Continuous arteriovenous haemofiltration and haemodifiltration in acute renal failure. Nephrol Dial Transplant 1988;2:181–186.
6   Hirasawa H, Sugai T, Ohtake Y, Sato HJ, Oda S, Shiga H, Aoe T: Energy metabolism and nutritional support in anuric multiple organ failure patients; in Tanaka T, Okada A (eds): Nutritional Support in Organ Failure, Amsterdam, Elsevier, 1990, pp 429–440.

7   Davenport A: Muscle weakness associated with prolonged continuous high flux haemofiltration. Intensive Care Med 1989;15:328–329.
8   Davenport A, Roberts NB: Amino acid losses during continuous high flux hemofiltration in the critically ill patient. Crit Care Med 1989;17:1010–1014.
9   Zobel G, Trop M, Muntean W, Ring E, Gleispach H: Anticoagulation for continuous arteriovenous hemolfiltration in children. Blood Purif 1988;6:90–95.

Dr. Hiroyuki Hirasawa, Department of Emergency and Critical Care Medicine, Chiba University School of Medicine, 1-8-1 Inohana, Chiba (Japan)

Sieberth HG, Mann H, Stummvoll HK (eds): Continuous Hemofiltration.
Contrib Nephrol. Basel, Karger, 1991, vol 93, pp 47–50

Continuous Arteriovenous Hemodialysis: Experience in Twenty-Six Intensive Care Patients

Erich Keller, Petra Reetze-Bonorden, Hans-Peter Lücking, Joachim Böhler, Peter Schollmeyer

Medical Clinic, Department of Nephrology, University of Freiburg, FRG

Continuous arteriovenous hemodialysis (CAVHD) combines the advantageous aspects of continuous arteriovenous hemofiltration (CAVH) and intermittent hemodialysis (HD) for the treatment of acute renal failure (ARF) in intensive care patients [1]. CAVHD adds diffusional transport processes to the continuous filtration by CAVH. It easily achieves control of uremia, fluid balance and electrolytes. We report the experience with CAVHD in 26 intensive care patients concerning technical problems, fluid removal, control of uremia, electrolytes, and patient outcome.

Patients and Methods

In 26 intensive-care patients (mean age 59 ± 14 years, range 30–72, 7 female) ARF occurred mostly due to septicemia (n = 16) or myocardial dysfunction (n = 5). In the other patients ARF was due to drug-induced liver and renal toxicity, malaria tropica, or pancreatitis. Two patients with polytrauma and multiorgan failure did not suffer from ARF but were chronically hemodialyzed before admittance. All patients were immobilized, needing mechanical respiration and parenteral nutrition.

Vascular access for CAVHD was achieved by percutaneous cannulation of the femoral artery and contralateral vein. Standard hemodialysis Shaldon catheters were connected via an arterial and venous line with a polyacrylonitrile plate dialyzer (Hospal®, AN69S, surface area 0.43 m^2). An infusion pump propelled 1 liter of dialysate (Schiwa®, Dialoc SH 04) per hour countercurrent to the blood flow through the dialyzer. To substitute ultrafiltrate, an electrolyte solution (Schiwa) was infused into the venous line. Anticoagulation was achieved by heparin infusion (300–600 IU/h) into the arterial line. When the ultrafiltration rate was repeatedly found below 100 ml/h, this was taken as a sign of clotting of the dialyzer and prompted replacement of the extracorporal system. Ultrafiltration was measured hourly and the substitution fluid was adapted to the clinical requirements.

Results

Total treatment time of all patients on CAVHD was 200 days, with a mean of 8 days per patient. The mean ultrafiltration rate measured 253 ± 118 ml/h, leading to approximately 6 liters ultrafiltrate per day. The

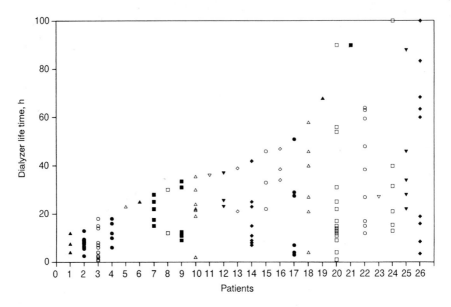

Fig. 1. The life span of the dialyzers varied markedly between and within the individual patients (n = 26).

mean life span of the dialyzer was 28 h (range 0.5–160 h), thus 5–6 dialyzers were used per patient, with marked interindividual differences (fig. 1). In some patients none of the dialyzers functioned adequately for more than 20 h (patients 1–4, fig. 1). Two of these patients had dissiminated intravascular coagulation, which may have caused frequent clotting of the filter. The life span of the plate did not correlate with (1) the partial thromboplastin time taken from the venous line (range 25–90 s); (2) hematocrit, or (3) serum protein concentration. However, there was a trend to short survival of filters with low mean daily blood pressures (fig. 2). At a mean arterial blood pressure below 70 mm Hg, no filter lasted longer than 18 h.

Start of renal replacement therapy in oliguric acute renal failure was instituted at a mean creatinine and urea concentration of 4.1 ± 2.3 and 156 ± 68 mg/dl, respectively. On the 3rd day creatinine measured 4.0 ± 2.1 mg/dl and urea was 146 ± 68 mg/dl, respectively. Subsequently, these parameters remained constant during the treatment despite anuria in most of these patients. The creatinine and the urea clearances due to CAVHD determined in a subgroup of 7 patients corresponded to the ultrafiltration/dialysate flow rate, being approximately 20 ml/min, because

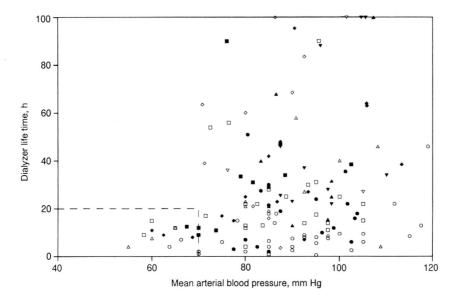

Fig. 2. The daily mean arterial blood pressure did not correlate with the dialyzers' life time. Note poor performance of dialyzers at mean arterial blood pressures below 70 mm Hg (dashed line).

urea and creatinine concentrations in dialysate/filtrate were >98% of plasma levels. None of the patients required additional intermittent hemodialysis. During CAVHD serum electrolytes were well controlled and serum potassium did not exceed 5.2 mmol/l. Despite an adequate control of uremia, only 4 of the patients survived. Two of them recovered from meningeal or pneumonial septicemia, one survived the complications of malaria tropica and one drug-induced liver and kidney failure. Major bleeding complications due to the arterial catheter or heparinisation were not observed.

Discussion

Since the institution of CAVH in the therapy of patients with ARF, several attempts have been made to increase the effectivity of this continuous renal replacement therapy [2]. Propelling dialysate through the filtrate compartment of the dialyzer has been described as one possibility to achieve this goal [1]. In comparison to CAVH, the different technical design of CAVHD requires a second infusion pump for the dialysate, handling of a dialysate volume of 24 liters/day. Calculations for fluid balance need to be modified accordingly.

A repeatedly found short survival of dialyzers in some of our patients is of major concern for adequacy of the treatment. The duration of adequate filter function appeared to be correlated mainly to technical problems like kinking of the catheters or extracorporal blood lines. The survival of the filter was, however, independent of the partial thromboplastin time or heparin doses. The lack of correlation of the dialyzers' life span to the mean daily blood pressure was an unexpected finding. The mean daily blood pressure taken from frequent measurements, however, may underestimate the meaning of short hypotensive episodes. Nevertheless, dialyzer life times were usually short when mean blood pressure was below 70 mm Hg. With disseminated intravascular coagulation the dialyzer life span may also remarkably be shortened as in patients 1 and 2 (fig. 1). The daily volume loss by CAVHD of approximately 6 liters allowed unrestricted parenteral nutrition and drug application. Despite adequate treatment of ARF with respect to urea, creatinine, electrolytes and volume control, the mortality of our patients was high. This indicates that in these severely ill hypercatabolic patients not ARF but the underlying disease determined the clinical outcome.

References

1   Geronemus R, Schneider N: Continuous arteriovenous hemodialysis: A new modality for treatment of acute renal failure. Trans Am Soc Artif Intern Organs 1984;30:610.
2   Kaplan A: The predilution mode for continuous arterioveneous hemofiltration; in Paganini P (ed): Acute Continuous Renal Replacement Therapy. Boston, Nijhoff, 1986, pp 143–172.

Dr. Erich Keller, Medizinische Universitätsklinik, Abteilung Innere Medizin IV, Dialysestation, Kilianstrasse 5, D–W–7800 Freiburg (FRG)

Sieberth HG, Mann H, Stummvoll HK (eds): Continuous Hemofiltration.
Contrib Nephrol. Basel, Karger, 1991, vol 93, pp 51–56

Decreased Mortality in Patients with Acute Renal Failure Undergoing Continuous Arteriovenous Hemodialysis

Brian R. McDonald, Ravindra L. Mehta[1]

University of California, San Diego UCSD Medical Center, San Diego, Calif., USA

Patients with acute renal failure (ARF) and multiple organ system failure (MOF) in the intensive-care unit (ICU) have mortality rates in excess of 80% [1]. The impact of renal replacement therapies in this group has been variable. More aggressive use of continuous replacement therapy may decrease patient mortality. We retrospectively analyzed the effect of two renal replacement therapies on the mortality of ICU patients with ARF.

Methods

We reviewed the charts of 42 ARF patients dialyzed in the medical, surgical and burn ICUs at UCSD Medical Center from December 1988 to March 1990. Patients received intermittent hemodialysis (IHD), continuous arteriovenous hemodialysis (CAVHD) or both therapies. Two periods were analyzed: (1) 8 months after initiation of a CAVHD program (December 88–July 89), and (2) 8 months thereafter (August 89–March 90).

IHD was performed using single-pass or sorbent dialysis machines. Cuprophane membranes with K_f 3.4–6.0 were used in all patients. Both acetate and bicarbonate dialysates were used at flow rates of 500 ml/min. Blood flow rates ranged from 250 to 300 ml/min. CAVHD was done using our modification of Geronemus and Schneider's technique [2] as previously described [3]. Hemodialysis was initially selected for hemodynamically stable patients [with mean arterial blood pressure (MAP) > 70 mm Hg]. CAVHD was initially performed in patients who failed the above criteria.

Results

Patient characteristics are depicted in table 1. IHD was performed initially in 20 patients with 10 crossovers to CAVHD. Of these, 8 switched

[1] We thank Maria Pascual, Petrea Monson and L. Taylor-Donald for their contributions.

Table 1. Characteristics of UCSD patients undergoing dialysis for ARF in ICU

Case No.	Age	Sex	Diagnosis	IHD	CAVHD	Both	Days on		Outcome
							IHD	CAVHD	
1	74	F	MI pulm. edema, ARF	+	−	−	2	−	died
2	33	M	IVDA, sepsis	−	−	+	4	3.5	died
3	49	M	S/P MVR, CHF	−	−	+	2	2.5	died
4	18	F	HUS, ARF	+	−	−	30	−	lived
5	29	M	MVA, fascitis, sepsis	−	+	+	7	5	lived
6	75	M	necrotic bowel sepsis	−	−	−	−	1	died
7	36	M	liver failure, sepsis	−	−	+	1	1	died
8	57	M	pulm. thromboendarterectomy	−	+	−	−	13.8	lived
9	61	M	liver failure, sepsis	−	+	−	−	2.7	died
10	50	M	TB, ARF	+	−	−	1	−	died
11	32	M	HIV, liver disease	−	−	+	1	4.2	died
12	39	M	pulm. thromboendarterectomy	−	+	−	−	2	died
13	70	M	ASCVD, CAD	+	−	−	2	−	died
14	38	F	S/P portocaval shunt	+	−	−	3	−	lived
15	35	M	liver failure GI bleed, sepsis	−	+	−	−	7.3	died
16	41	M	perirectal abcess, sepsis	−	+	−	−	5.1	died
17	63	F	S/P whipple, sepsis	−	−	+	2	1.7	died
18	43	F	pancreatitis, ARDS	−	−	+	1	10.7	died
19	62	M	S/P nephrectomy, sepsis, ARDS	+	+	−	−	38.6	died[a]
20	65	M	lymphoma, sepsis, ARF	−	−	−	1	−	died
21	29	F	trauma, MVA, sepsis	−	+	−	−	1.4	died
22	59	M	IVDA, liver failure, sepsis	−	+	−	−	1.4	died
23	81	F	trauma (MVA)	−	+	−	−	5.3	died

24	49	F	liver failure	+	−	−	−	3.9	died
25	35	M	IVDA, SBE, ARF	−	+	−	3	−	died
26	43	M	45% TBSA burn	+	−	−	−	20	died
27	44	M	liver failure	+	−	−	−	11	died
28	57	M	pulm. thromboendarterectomy	+	−	−	−	1	died
29	27	M	95% TBSA burn	+	−	−	−	16	lived
30	27	M	trauma, sepsis	+	−	−	−	0.5	died
31	32	F	cancer, sepsis	−	−	−	−	1	died
32	23	M	drowning	+	−	−	−	4	died
33	36	M	S/P portocaval shunt	−	+	−	50	−	died
34	43	M	head injury, sepsis	+	−	−	−	4	lived
35	54	F	cancer, sepsis	−	−	+	19	8	died
36	23	M	head injury, sepsis	−	−	+	23	10	lived
37	25	M	trauma, sepsis	+	−	−	−	6	died
38	40	M	cancer, aplasia	+	−	−	−	0.5	died
39	60	F	lymphoma, sepsis, ARF	−	+	−	13	−	lived
40	75	M	cryoglobulinemia, sepsis	−	−	+	2	12	died
41	50	M	S/P portocaval shunt, sepsis	−	+	−	9	−	died
42	42	F	postoperative sepsis	+	−	−	−	9	lived

MI = Myocardial infarction; pulm. = pulmonary; IVDA = intravenous drug abuse; S/P = status post; MVR = mitral valve replacement; CHF = congestive heart failure; HUS = hemolytic uremic syndrome; MVA = motor vehicle accident; TB = tuberculosis; HIV = human immunodeficiency virus; ASCVD = atherosclerotic cardiovascular disease; CAD = coronary artery disease; GI = gastrointestinal; ARDS = adult respiratory distress syndrome; SBE = subacute bacterial endocarditis; TBSA = total body surface area.

a Case 19: Patient was discharged from hospital and died at home.

Table 2. Severity of illness at onset of dialytic support

	Period 1			Period 2		
	IHD	IHD-CAVHD	CAVHD	IHD	IHD-CAVHD	CAVHD
>2 Organ systems failing	4 (67)	7 (100)	11 (100)	3 (75)	3 (100)	8 (72.7)
Ventilator-dependent	4 (67)	7 (100)	11 (100)	2 (66.7)	3 (100)	11 (100)
MAP < 70 mm Hg[a]	1 (16.7)	6 (85.7)	8 (72.7)	0 (–)	1 (33.3)	6 (54.5)

Figures in parentheses are percentages.
[a] IHD 1 vs. CAVHD 1: $p = 0.05$; IHD 2 vs. CAVHD 2: $p = 0.109$; IHD 2 vs. IHD-CAVHD 1: $p = 0.029$; IHD 1 vs. IHD-CAVHD 2: $p = 0.429$.

because of hemodynamic instability, and 2 had poor volume and solute control on IHD. 22 patients had CAVHD initially. Two CAVHD patients also received IHD; 1 required IHD after transfer from the ICU (case 8), while another transiently required it to allow femoral arterial access recovery (case 19). Mean numbers of treatments were 8.8 for all patients on IHD, and 6.6 treatment days for CAVHD. Severity of illness as evidenced by hypotension (MAP < 70), ventilator dependence and MOF is shown in table 2. There was no significant difference in severity of illness in the various groups from period 1 to period 2. However, in period 1, 16.7% of IHD patients had hypotension versus 72.7% CAVHD patients ($p = 0.05$) as compared to 0% (IHD) and 54.5% (CAVHD) in period 2 ($p = 0.109$). All CAVHD patients in period 1 had MOF versus the 67% IHD patients who had >2 MOF.

Detailed nutritional information was available in 8 patients in period 2. Two patients received IHD, 4 CAVHD and 2 were on both. Daily calculations of protein and caloric intake were done on these patients and the actual intake was expressed as a percentage of the prescribed nutritional goal. The results are shown in table 3. Patient mortality during this study is outlined in table 4.

Discussion

Although it appears from published studies [4] that CAVH and CAVHD are more efficacious and better tolerated than IHD in seriously ill patients, critical evaluation of these techniques in comparison with IHD has not been performed. Paganini [5] reported a series of ARF patients treated with dialysis: 19% underwent continuous therapy alone (slow continuous ultrafiltration, continuous arteriovenous hemofiltration, CAVHD); 48% had combined continuous therapy and IHD, and 33%

Table 3. Percentage of nutritional goals achieved with IHD versus CAVHD

	n	Kilocalorie	Protein intake
IHD	4	87.5 (6.7)	77.7 (8.83)
CAVHD	6	117.5 (6.4)	112.7 (3.02)

Results represent actual intake expressed as percentage of prescribed intake and are means with SEM given in parentheses.
IHD versus CAVHD: kilocalorie, $p = 0.012$; protein intake, $p = 0.02$.

Table 4. Decrease in patient mortality

	Period 1		Period 2		Change %
	n	mortality %	n	mortality %	
IHD	6	67	4	75	+12
IHD-CAVHD	7	86	3	67	−22
CAVHD	11	91	11	73	−20
Total	24	85	18	72	−13

received IHD alone. 92% of those on continuous therapy had MOF, compared to 80% in the combined group and 40% in the IHD group. Overall mortality was similar in all 3 groups and ranged from 76% in the combined group to 81% in the IHD group.

We also restrospectively analyzed the effect of CAVHD and IHD on the mortality of ARF patients in the ICU. We postulated that more aggressive use of continuous therapies could affect patient survival and we reviewed the effects of a CAVHD program over a 16-month period.

We found a decline in mortality in patients started on CAVHD or switched to CAVHD from IHD. A number of factors may account for this decrease. In the initial 8 months the CAVHD program was being established and CAVHD was used predominantly in hemodynamically unstable patients who would not tolerate IHD. This is evidenced by the greater incidence of hypotension in the CAVHD group and the IHD-CAVHD group in period 1. In the second 8 months, CAVHD was a more accepted modality and was used in preference to IHD. A second factor is probably the improved nutrition since fluid management is easier and nutritional goals were more easily achieved because of the glucose contribution from the dialysate in CAVHD patients. Thirdly, our staff became more familiar and proficient with CAVHD during the latter study period.

Our numbers are small and do not permit statistical comparison, but show a trend to better outcomes. We believe that CAVHD is preferable to IHD in treating ARF in the ICU setting and we are currently conducting a prospective randomized trial to further assess the relative efficacy of these two therapies.

References

1   Cameron JS: Acute renal failure: The continuing challenge. Q J Med 1986;234:977.
2   Geronemus R, Schneider N: Continuous arteriovenous hemodialysis: A new modality for the treatment of acute renal failure. ASAIO J 1984;30:610.
3   Mehta RL, McDonald BR, Aguilar MM, Ward DM: Regional citrate anticoagulation for continuous arteriovenous hemodialysis (CAVHD) in critically ill patients. Kidney Int 1990;38:976–981.
4   Gibney RTN, Stollery DE, Lefebvre RE, Sharun CJ, Chan P: Continuous arteriovenous hemodialysis: An alternative therapy for acute renal failure associated with critical illness. Can Med Assoc J 1988;139:861–866.
5   Paganini EP: Slow continuous hemofiltration and slow continuous ultrafiltration. AS-AIO J 1988;34:63–66.

Dr. Ravindra L. Mehta, University of California, San Diego, UCSD Medical Center, H–781D, 225 Dickinson, San Diego, CA 92103 (USA)

Sieberth HG, Mann H, Stummvoll HK (eds): Continuous Hemofiltration.
Contrib Nephrol. Basel, Karger, 1991, vol 93, pp 57–60

Outcome in Critically Ill Patients with Acute Renal Failure Treated by Continuous Hemofiltration

Gérald Keusch, Pia Schreier, Ulrich Binswanger

Section of Nephrology, Department of Internal Medicine, University Hospital, Zurich, Switzerland

Severe illness associated with acute renal failure (ARF) includes a mortality rate of approximately 50% which changed little over the last years [1, 2]. Patients who require renal replacement therapy during intensive care run an even higher risk with a mortality rate of 65 – 75% [3, 4]. Continuous hemofiltration (CHF) as a renal replacement therapy has some advantages and is especially suited for critically ill and hemodynamically unstable patients. It permits accurate control of fluid balance, adequate nutritional support and adequate control of uremia. This study deals with the clinical outcome of 49 critically ill patients with ARF treated by CHF.

Patients and Methods

Patients. During the time period from January 1984 through February 1988, 49 patients (M:F = 37:12) with ARF were treated by spontaneous arteriovenous or pump-assisted venovenous hemofiltration at our hospital. The mean age was 53 ± 16 (SD) years (range 22 – 76). Prior to hemofiltration the serum creatinine was $498 \pm 271 \, \mu mol/l$, the serum urea, $31 \pm 15 \, mmol/l$, and the serum potassium, $4.74 \pm 0.84 \, mmol/l$ of the patients, 28 were oliguric or anuric, 37 required mechanical ventilation, 16 had adult respiratory distress syndrome (ARDS), 43 required some form of vasopressor support and 28 had septicemia. The causes of ARF are shown in table 1.

Methods. Arteriovenous CHF was performed as originally described in 36 patients with femoral vessel catheters. In 13 patients pump-assisted venovenous CHF was performed by a double-lumen subclavian catheter. Blood was pumped using a roller pump at $100 \, ml \cdot min^{-1}$ through a polyamide hollow-fiber membrane filter (Gambro FH55 or 66). Anticoagulation of the extracorporeal circuit was achieved using a bolus dose of $1,000 – 2,000 \, IU$ of heparin followed by a constant infusion in the arterial line in the range of $300 – 1,000 \, IU/h$. In 7 patients with a thrombocytopenia of $4 – 31 \times 10^3/\mu l$ no continuous heparin infusion was given. The replacement fluid (potassium-free Ringer's lactate solution) was administered in 21 patients in a postdilution mode and in 28 patients in a predilution mode.

Table 1. Causes of ARF

Cause of ARF	Number of patients
Postoperative complication	27
Cardiac surgery	7
Abdominal aortic surgery	8
Abdominal surgery	9
Other surgical interventions	3
Multiple traumatic lesions	8
Major burns	2
Internal medical causes	12
Septicemia	7
Hemolytic-uremic syndrome	3
Hemorrhagic shock	1
Hepatorenal syndrome	1

Table 2. Outcome of patients with ARF treated by CHF

Cause of ARF	Number of patients		
	total	survived	died
Postoperative complication	27	10	17
Multiple traumatic lesions	8	2	6
Major burns	2	1	1
Internal medical causes	12	5	7
Total	49	18 (37%)	31 (63%)

Results

While 20 patients survived their episode of ARF only 18 patients (37%) were discharged alive from the hospital. The overall mortality rate was 63% and was not different in the various groups of patients (table 2). The survival rate in patients with ARF suffering from multiple traumatic lesions was slightly improved from 16 to 25% when compared to patients treated from 1976 to 1981 by intermittent hemodialysis at our hospital. The cause of death was related to septicemia in 13 patients, to multiorgan failure and septicemia in 8, to cardiovascular failure in 9 and to hepatic failure in 1. Septicemia complicating ARF prior to CHF treatment was more frequent in patients who died (21 out of 31) than in survivors (7 out of 18). This difference is statistically significant at $p < 0.05$ by χ^2 analysis. No difference in age, sex ratio, frequency of artificial ventilation, ARDS, vasopressor support and oliguria/anuria could be demonstrated between survivors and nonsurvivors. The mean duration of CHF treatment was 12.4 ± 7.9 days (range 3 – 41). Complication related to vascular access occurred in 3 patients: 1 femoral artery aneurysm at the site of femoral arterial puncture requiring surgical intervention; 1 femoral arteriovenous fistula, and 1 ischemic syndrome of the leg at the site of cannulation. Mild bleeding was seen in 4 patients, 1 of whom had disseminated intravascular coagulation and 3 thrombocytopenia ($17 - 39 \times 10^3/\mu l$). None of these complications were fatal.

Discussion

The total survival rate of 37% in this study in patients with ARF treated by CHF is comparable to other reports [5, 6]. Nevertheless, 63% of the patients still died during their acute illness despite good control of uremia. As in most other series septicemia was a major predictor of poor outcome. The presence of septicemia markedly increased mortality to as high as 70 – 90% in some studies [7, 8]. Sepsis has also been identified as the direct cause of death in 42% of our patients. Whether ARF itself predisposes the patient to sepsis or whether the clinical setting in which ARF occurs increases the risk of sepsis cannot be answered. Until we can deal with infection more effectively it is unlikely that mortality will fall to any significant extent. In addition, it has been suggested that the lack of improvement in survival may reflect a changing character of patients who present with ARF. Over time the population with ARF may have been skewed toward the older, sicker patient, who is more likely to have multiorgan failure [9]. Control of uremia by itself will not necessarily lead to any improvement in patient survival, and presumedly the outcome is predominantly influenced by the severity of the initial injury or illness.

References

1   Balslov JT, Jorgensen HE: A survey of 499 patients with acute anuric renal insufficiency. Am J Med 1963;34:753–764.
2   Bullock ML, Umen AJ, Finkelstein M, Keane WF: The assessment of risk factors in 462 patients with acute renal failure. Am J Kidney Dis 1985;5:97–103.
3   Crowin HL, Teplick RS, Schreiber MJ, Fang LST, Bonventre JV, Coggins CH: Prediction of outcome in acute renal failure. Am J Nephrol 1987;7:8–12.
4   Lohr JW, McFarlane MJ, Grantham JJ: A clinical index to predict survival in acute renal failure requiring dialysis. Am J Kidney Dis 1988;11:254–259.
5   Weiss L, Danielson BG, Wikström B, Hestrand U, Wahlberg J: Continuous arteriovenous hemofiltration in the treatment of 100 critically ill patients with acute renal failure: Report on clinical outcome and nutritional aspects. Clin Nephrol 1989;31:184–189.
6   Wendon J, Smithies M, Sheppard M, Bullen K, Tinker J, Bihari D: Continuous high volume venous-venous hemofiltration in acute renal failure. Intensive Care Med 1989;15:358–363.

7   Back SM, Makabali GG, Shoemaker WC: Clinical determinants of survival from
     postoperative renal failure. Surg Gynecol Obstet 1975;140:685–689.
8   Beaman M, Turney JH, Roger RSC, McGonigle RSJ, Adu D, Michael J: Changing
     pattern of acute renal failure. Q J Med 1987;62:15–23.
9   Butkus DE: Persistent high mortality in acute renal failure: Are we asking the right
     questions? Arch Intern Med 1983;143:209–212.

Gérald Keusch, MD, Section of Nephrology, Department of Internal Medicine,
University Hospital, Rämistrasse 100, CH–8091 Zürich (Switzerland)

Sieberth HG, Mann H, Stummvoll HK (eds): Continuous Hemofiltration.
Contrib Nephrol. Basel, Karger, 1991, vol 93, pp 61–64

Continuous Arteriovenous Hemodialysis and Hemofiltration in Acute Renal Failure: Comparison of Uremic Control

Abdelmoniem A. Alarabi, Björn Wikström, Bo G. Danielson

Department of Internal Medicine, University Hospital, Uppsala, Sweden

Continuous arteriovenous hemofiltration (CAVH) [1] has been widely used for the treatment of acute renal failure (ARF) in intensive-care patients with multiorgan failure and cardiovascular instability [2]. In our center, CAVH has been considered as the treatment of choice for ARF since 1982. During severe hypercatabolism control still has been a problem. Therefore, machine hemofiltration is needed in addition to CAVH. Recently, continuous arteriovenous hemodialysis (CAVHD) has been recommended for treatment in severely hypercatabolic patients [3]. To introduce CAVHD in our center for such patients and as an alternative to CAVH, this prospective study was performed comparing the efficiency of each modality in uremic control.

Materials and Methods

Thirteen intensive-care patients (8 males and 5 females) with ARF were included in the study. Mean age was 60 years (average 41 – 74 years). The ARF causes were medical ($n = 8$), post cardiac surgery ($n = 2$), post general surgery ($n = 2$) and major burns ($n = 1$). All patients were on mechanical respiration and vasopressor/inotropic drugs. Mean systolic blood pressure was 90 mm Hg (range 50 – 110 mm Hg). A 72-hour protocol was used starting with either CAVHD or CAVH in a randomized cross-over fashion every 24 h. Blood samples were tested every 8 h, following a pretreatment sample for urea, creatinine, glucose, electrolytes, hematocrit and partial thromboplastin time (PTT).

Both CAVH and CAVHD were performed with extracorporeal circuits as described previously [1, 3]. A polysulfone filter (Amicon D30) was used in this study. Hemofiltration solution SH23 (SCHI-WA, Glandorf, FRG), was used as dialysate and substitution fluid (it contains: Na, 142 mmol/l; Ca, 1.75 mmol/l; Mg, 0.5 mmol/l; K, 1 mmol/l; Cl, 103 mmol/l; lactate, 44.5 mmol/l). The dialysate flow rate was kept at 15 ml/min during CAVHD. It was infused in a counter-current direction to the arterial blood flow. The dialysate and ultrafiltration (UF) bag was kept at the level of the hemofilter during CAVHD to minimize UF unless otherwise indicated. The UF range during CAVH was 600 – 750 ml/h.

For vascular access the Buselmeier shunt was used in 9 patients and femoral vessel cannulation in 4 patients. Heparin was given at the start of treatment in a bolus dose of

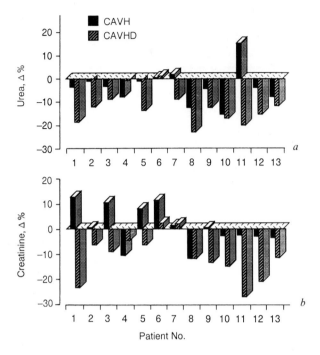

Fig. 1. Effects of CAVH and CAVHD treatments on the serum urea *(a)* and creatinine *(b)* levels in individual patients.

Table 1. Effect of CAVH and CAVHD on serum urea and creatinine levels (mean ± SD)

Treatment	Serum urea mmol/l	Δ %	Serum creatinine μmol/l	Δ %	UF volume l/24 h
CAVH, start	30 ± 12		405 ± 173		
		−1 ± 9		−1 ± 8	14 ± 5.6
CAVH, steady state	29 ± 12		401 ± 158		
CAVHD, start	32 ± 13		432 ± 165		
		−10 ± 10		−11 ± 9	8 ± 2.8
CAVHD, steady state	28 ± 12		387 ± 153		

1,000 – 4,000 IU and then as an infusion (10 – 15 IU/kg body weight) in order to keep the PTT at 40 – 100 s.

Nutritional fluids were given intravenously (amino acids, 0.8 – 1.2 g/kg body weight/day; carbohydrates, 1,500 – 3,000 kcal/day). In the diabetic patients soluble insulin was usually added to the infusion solution of glucose (30%).

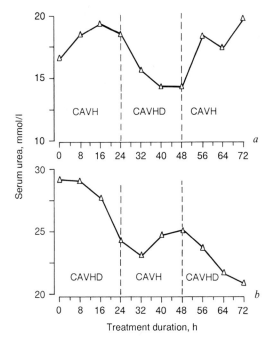

Fig. 2. Serum urea profiles during CAVH and CAVHD in 2 patients *(a* and *b).*

Results

The ranges of the pretreatment serum urea and creatinine levels were 15 – 56 mmol/l and 295 – 679 μmol/l, respectively (in 9 patients the serum urea range was 31 – 56 mmol/l). This indicates that the majority of these patients were severely hypercatabolic. Average daily urine output was 0 – 450 ml.

The effect of CAVH or CAVHD on serum urea and creatinine levels was evaluated as a difference ($\Delta\%$) during each treatment session (table 1, fig. 1). A significant difference was noted during CAVHD but not during CAVH ($p < 0.01$ for both urea and creatinine). This effect is clearly illustrated in figure 2 for 2 patients, indicating that CAVHD is more effective than CAVH for removal of urea. The net UF rate during CAVHD was approximately 50% of that during CAVH.

Discussion

Both CAVH and CAVHD are now widely used for the treatment of ARF. Recent comparative studies between CAVH and CAVHD in man and in mathematical models [4 – 7] showed a significant effect of CAVHD over CAVH concerning the elimination of small-molecular-weight solutes.

This is in agreement with our results. Despite this fact, in a few patients, the blood urea was rising even during CAVHD, which was attributed to the relatively low dialysate flow rate (15 ml/min) used in this study. In our view, CAVHD is technically as simple as CAVH with less frequency of filter clotting. It could be considered as a treatment of choice for ARF in severe hypercatabolic states.

References
1   Kramer P, Kaufhold G, Gröne HJ, Wigger W, Rieger J, Matthaei D: Management of anuric intensive care patients with arteriovenous hemofiltration. Int J Artif Organs 1980;3:225–230.
2   Wheeler DC, Feehaly J, Walls J: High risk acute renal failure. Q J Med 1986;61:977–984.
3   Geronemus R, Schneider N: Continuous arteriovenous hemodialysis (CAVHD): A new modality for treatment of acute renal failure. Trans Am Soc Artif Intern Organs 1984;30:610–613.
4   Raja R, Kramer P, Goldstein S, Caruana R, Lerner A: Comparison of continuous arteriovenous hemofiltration and continuous arteriovenous hemodialysis in critically ill patients. Trans Am Soc Artif Intern Organs 1986;32:435–436.
5   Sigler MH, Teehan BP: Solute transport in continuous arteriovenous hemodialysis: A new treatment for acute renal failure. Kidney Int 1987;32:562–571.
6   Schneider NS, Geronemus RP: Continuous arteriovenous hemodialysis. Kidney Int 1988;33(suppl 24):159–162.
7   Pallone TL, Hyver S, Petersen J: The simulation of continuous arteriovenous hemodialysis with a mathematical model. Kidney Int 1989;35:125–133.

Dr. Abdelmoniem A. Alarabi, Department of Internal Medicine,
University Hospital, S–751 85 Uppsala (Sweden)

Cardiac and Pulmonary Diseases

Sieberth HG, Mann H, Stummvoll HK (eds): Continuous Hemofiltration.
Contrib Nephrol. Basel, Karger, 1991, vol 93, pp 65–70

Influence of Ultrafiltration/Hemofiltration on Extravascular Lung Water

Anton N. Laggner, Wilfred Druml, Kurt Lenz, Bruno Schneeweiss,
Georg Grimm

First Department of Medicine, University of Vienna, Austria

Pulmonary edema is characterized by an increase of extravascular lung water (EVLW) which is caused either by elevated hydrostatic microvascular pressure or impaired capillary permeability. The clinical conditions in which hydrostatic pulmonary edema develops are mainly hypervolemia and left ventricular failure. Therefore, this type of pulmonary edema is often referred to as cardiogenic pulmonary edema (CPE). An increase in microvascular permeability develops under several conditions, i.e. sepsis, pneumonia, disseminated intravascular coagulation, intoxications, and results in severe impairment of pulmonary gas exchange. Therefore, this type of pulmonary edema is often referred to as adult respiratory distress syndrome (ARDS).

The use of ultrafiltration (UF) and/or hemofiltration (HF) has been suggested for treatment of both CPE and ARDS and more or less beneficial effects have been published. In this paper we report our experience on the influence of UF/HF on EVLW in both CPE and ARDS.

Material and Methods

The clinical characteristics of patients with CPE are listed in table 1. CPE was defined by an elevated EVLW and a pulmonary artery wedge pressure (PCWP) > 18 mm Hg [1]. The clinical characteristics of patients with ARDS are listed in table 2. ARDS was defined by an elevated EVLW, a PCWP ≤ 18 mm Hg, and a cardiac index (CI) > 3 liters/min/m² [2].

Before UF/HF, an arterial catheter (Femoral Artery Lung Water Catheter 96–020-5F, Edwards, USA) was introduced into the femoral artery and a flow-directed pulmonary artery catheter was advanced under pressure control, until a typical wedge tracing was obtained. PCWP and central venous pressure (CVP) were recorded by a Hewlett-Packard transducer 1290 A (with the midaxillary line as zero reference) and a Hewlett-Packard multichannel recorder. Cardiac output (CO) was determined by the thermodilution method (Hewlett-Packard Cardiac Output Module 78231 C). EVLW was measured by the thermal dye technique using a lung water computer (9310, Edwards, USA). The method and its reproducibility has been described extensively [3].

Table 1. Number (No.), initials (I), sex (S), age (A), underlying disorder, outcome, fluid balance (ml) and duration of HF (h) of 8 patients with CPE

No.	I	S	A	Underlying disorder	Outcome	UF/HF	
						balance	duration
1	EE	f	34	hepatorenal syndrome	alive	−2,500	6
2	NF	m	59	AMI, acute renal failure	alive	−2,500	3
3	KF	m	59	renal failure, apoplexia	died	−1,300	3
4	BF	m	49	acute renal failure	alive	−2,500	4
5	KF	m	39	renal failure	alive	−2,500	4
6	EW	m	62	congestive CMP	alive	−2,500	6
7	MA	f	60	renal failure	died	−2,500	4
8	IH	m	59	acute renal failure, AMI	alive	−8,140	16

Table 2. Number (No.), initials (I), sex (S), age (A), underlying disorder, outcome, fluid balance (ml) and duration of HF (h) of 9 patients with ARDS

No.	I	S	A	Underlying disorder	Outcome	UF/HF	
						balance	duration
1	MI	f	21	lupus erythematodes	alive	−9,450	29
2	HH	m	40	Goodpasture's syndrome	died	−4,050	12
3	BM	m	40	Wegener's granulomatosis	alive	−10,000	17
4	DH	m	39	intoxication (chlorate)	died	−2,000	3
5	BL	f	48	sepsis, liver cirrhosis	died	−2,000	4
6	AL	f	75	sepsis, liver cirrhosis	died	−1,500	3
7	SF	m	52	intoxication (TCE)	alive	−4,000	16
8	KE	f	33	septic abortion	died	−2,900	29
9	HE	f	39	pneumonia, liver cirrhosis	died	−2,400	24

Blood samples for blood gas analysis and oximetry (IL 1303, IL Co-oxymeter 282, Instrumentation Laboratories, USA) from arterial and mixed venous blood were drawn under anaerobic conditions into 5-ml syringes. For evaluation of pulmonary oxygenation, arterial oxygen partial pressure (PaO_2) was divided by the fraction of inspired oxygen (FiO_2). Venous admixture (Q_s/Q_t) and oxygen delivery (DO_2) were calculated according to standard formulas. Colloid-osmotic pressure (COP) was measured by a mercury calibrated, membrane transducer system (Oncometer BMT 921, Thomae FRG). For pump-driven (HD 104 and HD 105, Braun, FRG) UF/HF (Hemofilter Amicon 20, FRG) a venovenous or arteriovenous access was used. Fluid replacement was performed with a specially designed electrolyte solution (Hämfl MD, Leopold, Austria). For statistical analysis the values before and after UF/HF were compared by Student's t test for paired data.

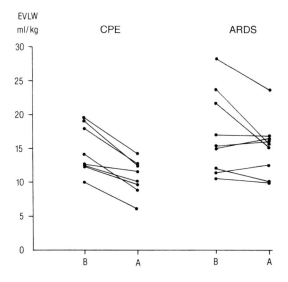

Fig. 1. Influence of CHF on EVLW in patients with CPE and ARDS. Values were obtained before (**B**) and after (**A**) UF/HF treatment.

Results

The influence of UF/HF on EVLW in patients with CPE and ARDS is documented in figure 1. The 8 patients with CPE showed a uniform decrease in EVLW from 15.4 ml/kg before to 12.3 ml/kg after UF/HF ($p < 0.05$). In ARDS, in 4 out of 9 patients only, a more than 15% reduction of EVLW was achieved. In this group, EVLW only slightly decreased (from 17.9 ± 5.5 ml/kg before to 15.8 ± 4.2 ml/kg after UF/HF). Hemodynamic and gas exchange parameters before and after UF/HF are listed in table 3. In patients with CPE a significant decrease in PCWP, CVP, Q_s/Q_t was accompanied by a significant increase in COP. In patients with ARDS a significant decrease in CO was accompanied by a decrease in DO_2. COP increased significantly.

Discussion

UF/HF have been advocated for reduction of EVLW in both CPE [4–9] and ARDS [10–15]. This beneficial effect has been attributed to an ultrafiltration-induced reduction of microvascular pressure, increased in intravascular COP, and the hemofiltration-induced elimination of middle molecular weight substances, which were considered responsible for development of ARDS [16].

Table 3. Hemodynamic and gas exchange parameters before and after UF/HF in patients with CPE and ARDS

	CPE (n = 8)		ARDS (n = 9)	
	before	after	before	after
PCWP, mm Hg	25 ± 5	18 ± 6*	14 ± 2	12 ± 2
CVP, mm Hg	12 ± 4	7 ± 4*	7 ± 3	$4 + 4$
CO, l/min	8.5 ± 2.0	8.5 ± 2.4	8.8 ± 2.9	6.0 ± 2.7*
PaO_2/FiO_2, mm Hg	290 ± 146	341 ± 93	95 ± 27	132 ± 79
Q_s/Q_t, %	27 ± 12	20 ± 10*	50 ± 10	34 ± 14*
DO_2, ml/min/m^2	555 ± 184	556 ± 176	492 ± 143	376 ± 163
COP, mm Hg	21.8 ± 3.9	23.2 ± 3.7*	20.1 ± 2.5	23.9 ± 5.7*

*$p < 0.05$.

In our study we found a significant reduction of EVLW in patients with CPE by UF/HF. In these patients the elevated microvascular pressure was lowered by UF/HF, thereby reducing fluid filtration rate. Additionally the UF/HF-induced increase in intravascular COP favored reabsorption of fluid from the extravascular to the intravascular compartment. These mechanisms seem to be responsible for the reduction of EVLW by UF/HF in patients with CPE.

In patients with ARDS, despite lowering microvascular pressures and significantly increasing COP, we were unable to demonstrate similar beneficial effects. Moreover, UF/HF adversely affected CO, which further impaired oxygen transport to the tissues. In ARDS pulmonary microvascular permeability is impaired. As hydrostatic pressure is primarily normal, UF/HF-induced reduction in microvascular pressure cannot be expected to lower fluid filtration rate as in CPE. Additionally the UF/HF-induced increase in intravascular COP may not favor reabsorption of fluid to the intravascular compartment, as due to the impaired permeability, a colloid osmotic pressure gradient cannot develop. These mechanisms seem to be responsible for the fact that UF/HF in ARDS was not as effective as in CPE. Moreover, the UF/HF-induced reduction in hydrostatic pressures lead to the nonbeneficial drop in cardiac output in ARDS.

Regarding our results, several objections have to be made. Both time (3–16 h in CPE patients and 3–29 h in ARDS patients) and net fluid balance ($-1,300$ to $-8,140$ ml in CPE and -1500 to $-10,000$ ml in ARDS patients) of HF/UF differed considerably between the individuals and we cannot predict the effect of a standard HF/UF regimen in both

CPE and ARDS. Additionally we cannot predict the effect of continuous HF (CHF) with positive net fluid balances. Gotloid et al. [12, 16] reported beneficial pulmonary effects of CHF even with positive net fluid balances in patients with sepsis and attributed these effects to the elimination of middle molecular weight substances.

In patients with CPE, UF/HF offers a means for reduction of EVLW without adversely affecting CO and oxygen delivery to the tissues. In patients with ARDS due to the underlying condition, the pulmonary effects of UF/HF are less beneficial. In these patients UF/HF sould be performed under close hemodynamic monitoring.

References

1 Sibbald WJ, Cunningham DR, Chin DN: Non-cardiac or cardiac pulmonary edema? A paractical approach to clinical differentiation in critically ill patients. Chest 1983;84:452–461.

2 Laggner AN, Lenz K, Grimm G, Sommer G, Gössinger H: Hämofiltration zur Reduktion des Lungenwassers beim ARDS? Schweiz Med Wochenschr 1987;117:445–449.

3 Laggner AN, Lenz K, Druml W, Kleinberger G: Reproducibility of thermal-dye lung water measurements by a lung water computer in critically ill patients. Crit Care Med 1987;15:606–608.

4 Coraim FJ, Coraim HP, Ebermann R, Stellwag FM: Acute respiratory failure after cardiac surgery: Clinical experience with the application of continuous arteriovenous hemofiltration. Crit Care Med 1986;14:714–718.

5 Fauchald P, Forfang K, Amlie J: An evaluation of ultrafiltration as treatment of therapy-resistant cardiac edema. Acta Med Scand 1986;219:47–51.

6 Magilligan D, Oyama C, Levin N: Interstitial and intraalveolar pulmonary edema-reversal by ultrafiltration (abstract). Crit Care Med 1981;9:257.

7 Oyama C, Levin N, Magilligan DJ Jr: Pulmonary edema: reversal by ultrafiltration. J Surg Res 1984;36:191–197.

8 Rimondini A, Cipolla CM, Della Bella P, Grazi S, Sisillo E, Susini G, Guazzi MD: Hemofiltration as short-term treatment for refractory congestive heart failure. Am J Med 1987;83:43–448.

9 Simpson IA, Rae AP, Gribben J, Boulton-Jones JM, Allison ME, Hutton I: Ultrafiltration in the management of refractory congestive heart failure. Br Heart J 1986;55:344–347.

10 Barckow D, Schirop T: Isolierte Ultrafiltration beim akuten Lungenversagen. Intensivmedizin 1983;20:213–216.

11 Lewis RM, Henning RJ, Besso J, Weil MH: Ultrafiltration for the treatment of adult respiratory distress syndrome. Heart Lung 1984;13:381–386.

12 Gotloib L, Barzilay E, Shustak A, Lev A: Sequential hemofiltration in nonoliguric high capillary permeability pulmonary edema of severe sepsis: preliminary report. Crit Care Med 1984;12:997–1000.

13 Gotloid L, Barzilay E, Shustak A, Waiss Z, Lev A: Hemofiltration in severe high microvascular permeability pulmonary edema secondary to rickettsial spotted fever. Resuscitation 1985;13:25–29.

14 Sivak ED, Tita J, Meden G, Ishigami M, Graves J, Kavlich J, Stowe NT, Magnusson MO: Effects of furosemide versus isolated ultrafiltration on extravascular lung water in oleic acid-induced pulmonary edema. Crit Care Med 1986;14:48–51.

15   Sznajder JI, Zucker AR, Wood LDH, Long GR: The effects of plasmapheresis and hemofiltration on canine acid aspiration pulmonary edema. Am Rev Resp Dis 1986;134:222–228.
16   Gotloid L, Barzilay E: The impact of using the artificial kidney as an artificial endocrine lung upon severe septic ARDS. Intensive Crit Care Dig 1986;5:3–5.

Anton N. Laggner, MD, First Department of Medicine, University of Vienna, Lazarettgasse 14, A–1090 Vienna (Austria)

Sieberth HG, Mann H, Stummvoll HK (eds): Continuous Hemofiltration.
Contrib Nephrol. Basel, Karger, 1991, vol 93, pp 71–75

Pathology of Multiple Organ Failure

B. Klosterhalfen, F.A. Offner, C.J. Kirkpatrick, C. Mittermayer

Institute of Pathology, Technical University of Aachen, RWTH, Aachen, FRG

Shock of varying origin, especially septic shock, is a common problem of modern critical-care medicine and closely related to multiple organ failure (MOF). Multiple organ systems can fail if the alterations lead to an inadequate perfusion of vital organs with subsequent disturbance of the metabolic steady state of the cells [1–5].

Organ Systems at Risk

The organ systems at risk for failure in critically ill individuals are numerous. At autopsy of MOF patients, alterations of nearly all organs can be verified. The cardiovascular, pulmonary and renal systems are the target organs most commonly associated with pathomorphological changes and are those most commonly recognized by the clinician to fail. Failure of the gastrointestinal tract is characterized by stress-related ulceration, with or without bleeding. Pancreatic failure, uncontrolled catabolism and disseminated intravascular coagulation are presumed in patients with altered clinical features and laboratory parameters, which may reflect a pancreatic disorder, substrate-metabolism abnormalities or a dysfunction of the normal hemostatic mechanisms of the coagulation cascade, respectively. Finally, disorientation that may proceed to coma in the critically ill patient suggests that even neurological failure may be a component of this syndrome.

Histological Findings in the Main Target Organs

Lung. The cardinal histological feature of the adult respiratory distress syndrome is the finding of leukocyte aggregates, together with platelet emboli and fibrin in the pulmonary arterioles. Fluid leaks from the capillaries into the interstitium of the lungs and then into the alveoli, which soon contain protein-rich hyaline membranes. Leukocytes gradually infiltrate the edematous interstitium from the blood, but the condition can be distinguished from pneumonia because white cells are not seen in the alveoli from the outset. Interstitial fibrosis often follows as a consequence of the permeability defects. The alveolar wall now can be 130 μm in thickness, that is of the order of 20 times more than that of the healthy lung (5–7 μm) [6].

Liver. The characteristic pathological microscopic findings of the shock liver are centrilobular necrosis, central vein and sinusoidal congestion, bile stasis, edema and hyperemia. These changes are maximal around the central vein, which is the effluent channel of the hepatic blood system with the lowest oxygen content. The cirrhotic liver is much more liable to oxygen deficits during the course of shock, and thus liver failure is the leading clinical and pathomorphologic correlation in these patients.

Kidney. The kidneys are major targets in severe shock, principally affecting the tubules at all levels of the nephron. The tubular lesions are referred to as acute tubular necrosis. The microscopic findings are characterized by widened tubules with defects of the tubular epithelium. The association of renal failure with failure of at least two other organ systems usually has a lethal outcome.

Heart. The target organ heart is affected in all forms of shock. Distinctive cardiac changes are subepicardial and subendocardial hemorrhages and areas of necrosis, as well as zonal lesions, called contraction band necrosis. The forms of necrosis range from isolated fiber ischemic lesions to larger areas of involvement comprising micro- or macroinfarcts.
Abacterial endocarditis or endocarditis verrucosa simplex are other typical macro- and microscopic findings in MOF [7].

Adrenal Glands. These glands react to all forms of stress and shock. The spectrum of change extends from lipid depletion to scattered necrosis of isolated cells in the cortex beginning in the zona reticularis and spreading in an outward fashion. Hemorrhages are common, especially in meningococcal sepsis, which often presents as the Waterhouse-Friderichsen syndrome, with necrosis and hemorrhage in both glands.

Gastrointestinal Tract. The intestine in shock may develop the pathomorphological features of a hemorrhagic gastroenteropathy. The blood circulation in the mucosa is almost selectively decreased, while the submucosa and muscularis propria are spared the decrease in blood supply. Thus, the preferential localization for intestinal tissue damage is the mucosa of the stomach, jejunum and ileum, in decreasing order of frequency. The colonic mucosa is rarely involved. Older patients are more often affected, especially if the superior mesenteric artery is partially or totally obliterated by arteriosclerosis. Often the damage is segmental, corresponding with the anatomical distribution of the intestinal vascular supply. The initial necrotizing process may end in a pseudomembranous enteritis.

Some authors regard the gut as a decisive motor or alternatively as source of MOF. Recent progress in the assay of endotoxin with the limulus test and immunohistochemistry has indicated that the intestine may be responsible for the irreversibility of shock. Permeability defects and later shock-induced tissue damage to the intestine allow intestinal bacteria or their products, endo- and ectotoxins, to penetrate the intestinal wall and to gain access to the blood circulation [8]. In many cases shock-induced lesions of the gut are probably responsible for setting MOF in motion and maintaining it.

Brain. The brain suffers so-called hypoxic encephalopathy, although brain lesions are rare. Occasionally, microscopic hemorrhages are seen, but patients who recover do not show neurological deficits. In severe cases, particularly in patients with cerebral atherosclerosis, hemorrhage and necrosis may appear in the overlapping region between the terminal distributions of major arteries.

With certain exceptions, the cellular and organ changes encountered in shock are reversible if the patient survives. Thus, regeneration in renal tubular cells, adrenocortical cells, hepatocytes and gastrointestinal mucosa may be complete. Loss of neurons in the brain and myocytes in the heart, as well as septal pulmonary fibrosis may constitute an irreversible tissue damage.

Role of the Endothelial Cell Layer

Alteration and damage of the endothelial cells at different vessel sites during the course of shock may play a key role in the development of MOF [9, 10]. The integrity of the vessel walls with special regard to the small venules and capillaries of the microcirculatory system guarantees an intact permeability barrier.

The first morphological alteration in the endothelial cells occurs only a few hours after onset of shock. The endothelial cells show apical cytoplasmic diverticula, a result of endothelial cell cytoplasmic swelling or vacuole formation. Microvesicles as a result of increased pinocytosis were detected in transmission electron micrographs. Especially endothelial cells of the smallest branches of the pulmonary artery and the heart valves are injured.

Various Mediators of Multiple Organ Failure

Prostaglandins. In the past 2 decades, prostacyclin and thromboxane received the greatest interest in septic shock research. Both prostacyclin and thromboxane are elevated in the plasma of septic shock patients, depending on the severity of sepsis. Prostacyclin has profound vasodilatory effects and inhibits platelet aggregation, whereas thromboxane is a microcirculatory vasoconstrictor and powerful aggregator of platelets. Prostacyclin has generally been viewed as a favorable prostaglandin by virtue of its vasodilatory effects, thromboxane on the other hand as being an adverse mediator in septic shock. The cellular and microvascular effects, as well as the role in pathogenesis in MOF, still need further research.

Interleukins and Tumor Necrosis Factor-α. Systemic release of interleukin-1 (IL-1) from macrophages may be stimulated during the course of septic shock by endotoxins or bacteria. First described as endogenous pyrogen or granulocytic pyrogen, IL-1 is a group of similar proteins that act on the hypothalamus to produce fever. In parallel, IL-1 stimulates the production of IL-6 responsible for the release of acute-phase proteins such as α_2-macroglobulin.

To add to the complexity, several lines of experimental evidence suggest that the production of prostaglandins, leukotrienes, platelet-activating factor (PAF), and IL-1 is signaled by the release of tumor necrosis factor-α (TNF-α) from monocytes and macrophages. Increased serum levels of TNF-α have been demonstrated in patients suffering from sepsis and in several animal models of endotoxic shock. TNF-α and IL-1 may play a key role in the pathogenesis of MOF.

PAF and Leukotrienes. PAF and leukotrienes (particularly LTE_4), presumably derived from neutrophils and endothelial cells, have been observed in numerous experimental animal models of septic shock, but their contribution to the clinical state remains unresolved.

Oxygen Radicals. Charged oxygen radicals have a very potent capability to irreversibly damage biological membranes. Normally, oxygen radicals are produced by activated neutrophils as part of the mechanism to eliminate phagocytized microorganisms. Degranulation of these neutrophils, perhaps secondary to complement activation, makes oxygen radicals a potent mediator of tissue damage. Inappropriate synthesis or release is the result of two principal mechanisms. First, activated neutrophils adherent to endothelial cells or other tissue cells produce oxygen radicals. Direct contact with the cells results in endothelial cell or tissue damage. A second mechanism for oxygen radicals to serve as a mediator of tissue damage can be identified as a consequence of cellular shock or hypoxia via activation of xanthine oxidase and degradation of adenine nucleotides, which results in hypoxanthine which is then oxidized via xanthine oxidase. The liberated radicals are then thought to mediate lipid peroxidation within the cell, thus causing cellular injury. Both visceral and particularly endothelial cells are vulnerable to this mechanism. Oxygen free radicals appear to play an essential role in the pathogenesis of MOF.

References

1 Carrico CJ, Meakins JL, Marshall JC, Fry D, Maier RV: Multiple-organ-failure syndrome. Arch Surg 1986;121:196–208.
2 McMenamy RH, Birkhahn R, Oswald G, Reed R, Rumph C, Vaidyanath N, Yu L, Cerra FB, Sorkness R, Border JR: Multiple systems organ failure. I. The basal state. J Trauma 1981;21:99–114.
3 Border J: Hypothesis: Sepsis, multiple systems organ failure, and the macrophage. Arch Surg 1988;123:285–286.
4 Fry D: Multiple systems organ failure. Surg Clin North Am 1988;68:107–122.
5 Neuhof H: Ursachen und Therapie von Organversagen: Mediatoren, ihr Stellenwert und therapeutische Implikation am Beispiel des septischen Patienten. Langenbecks Arch Chir 1987;372:43–47.
6 Riede UN, Joachim H, Hassenstein J, Costabel U, Sandritter W, Augustin P, Mittermayer C: The pulmonary air-blood barrier of human shock lungs: A clinical, ultrastructural and morphometric study. Pathol Res Pract 1978;162:41–72.
7 Klosterhalfen B, Fehrenbach T, Kirkpatrick CJ, Mittermayer C: Abacterial endocarditis due to endotoxemia. Intensive Care Med 1990;16:19.
8 Deitch EA, Winterton J, Berg R: The gut as a portal of entry for bacteria: Role of protein malnutrition. Ann Surg 1987;205:681–692.
9 Schoeffel U, Shiga J, Mittermayer C: The proliferation-inhibiting effect of endotoxin on human endothelial cells in culture and its possible implication in states of shock. Circ Shock 1982;9:499–508.
10 Rixen H, Klosterhalfen B, Pennartz G, Teniz A, Schulz M, Kirkpatrick CJ: Injury to endothelial cells and decrease in proliferation during the course of septic shock. Intensive Care Med 1990;16:34.

Dr. B. Klosterhalfen, Institute of Pathology, RWTH Aachen, Pauwelsstrasse 30, D–W–5100 Aachen (FRG)

Sieberth HG, Mann H, Stummvoll HK (eds): Continuous Hemofiltration.
Contrib Nephrol. Basel, Karger, 1991, vol 93, pp 76–78

Continuous Venovenous Hemodialysis after Cardiac Surgery

O. Bastien, C. Saroul, C. Hercule, M. George, S. Estanove

Département d'Anesthésie-Réanimation, Hôpital Cardiologique, Lyon, France

Acute renal failure (ARF) after cardiac surgery is often related to low cardiac output. High mortality rate (sometimes more than 70% [1]) could be associated with cardiac instability. The aim of the study was to test this hypothesis and compare conventional hemodialysis (CH) with continuous venovenous hemodialysis (CVVHD).

Method and Patients

All patients since 1986, with ARF, except chronic or obstructive renal disease, were included. The CH group used the standard procedure of hemodialysis, including increase of inotropic support if necessary, and generally bicarbonate as the dialysate buffer. The CVVHD group used a low blood flow rate (50 ml/min) and a closed sterile dialysis fluid (Hospal: 1 liter/h) through a polyacrylonitrile membrane (AN 69 Hospal). The vascular access was a double lumen venous catheter to preserve femoral arteries specially for surgical procedures (aortic dissection, bypass). There was no randomization by reason of increasing development of CVVHD since 1988, and so the groups were chronologic. The study examines etiology, Apache II severity score, mortality rate of the two groups. Hemodynamic stability during CVVHD without change of inotropic therapy has been tested at T_0 (before dialysis), T_1 (1/4 h), T_2 (1 h), T_3 (24 h), using ejection fraction and volumetric Swan-Ganz catheter (REF 1 Edwards). Statistics used χ^2 test with Yates correction, Student's test for quantitative data, and ANOVA (Newman-Keuls test) for repeated measurements.

Results

The CH group included 32 patients and the CVVHD group 34. They were similar concerning etiology, age, severity score and creatinine level (table 1). ARF with preserved diuresis seems to have a better prognosis and mortality decreases from 87% (anuric) to 44% ($p < 0.05$). The number of patients with preserved diuresis was similar between the groups (9 in CH versus 7 in CVVHD). Hemodynamic stability during CVVHD was confirmed (table 2), without any change of preload, cardiac index or systemic blood pressure.

Table 1. CH and CVVHD population studied

	CH	CVVHD
Etiology		
Coronary disease	5	1
Valvular surgery	9	14
Aortic disease	5	7
Transplantation	13	12
Mean age, years	54 ± 13	60 ± 12
Apache II	19.8 ± 5	22.5 ± 7
Azotemia, mmol/l	46.7 ± 13	35 ± 14 ($p < 0.05$)
Creatinine, μmol/l	511 ± 253	447 ± 182
Mortality, %	75	50

Table 2. Hemodynamic data

	T_0	T_1	T_2	T_3
MAP, mm Hg	75 ± 11	72 ± 8	75 ± 9	78 ± 15
PAOP, mm Hg	18 ± 6	16 ± 8	17 ± 7	17 ± 8
CI, l/min/m²	2.92 ± 0.5	2.80 ± 0.7	2.97 ± 0.7	2.93 ± 0.5
RVEF, %	0.40 ± 0.1	0.37 ± 0.08	0.38 ± 0.11	0.43 ± 0.1
EDVI, ml/m²	63 ± 16	62 ± 16	63 ± 15	74 ± 17

MAP = Mean arterial pressure; PAOP = pulmonary artery occlusive pressure; CI = cardiac index; RVEF = right ventricular ejection fraction; EDVI = end-diastolic volume index. T_0 = Before dialysis; $T_1 = \frac{1}{4}$ h, $T_2 = 1$ h, $T_3 = 24$ h during CVVHD.

Discussion

In spite of a daily ultrafiltration of more than 4 liters ($4,902 \pm 2,107$ ml) and correction of overhydration (weight $0 = 64.1 \pm 12$ versus weight $1 = 62.5 \pm 12$ kg), the right and left ventricular preload measured by right atrial pressure, right end-diastolic volume index (EDVI) and pulmonary artery occlusive pressure (PAOP) may be preserved. Non-randomized but comparative groups seem to have a different prognosis. Despite multifactorial factors, systemic and renal hemodynamic effects should be determinant [2]. The mortality rate of 50% seems improved by this stability.

Using no deleterious type of hemodialysis could probably authorize earlier management of ARF, as it seems with a lower urea level in the CVVHD group. According to other authors [3], oliguric renal failure increases mortality risk. Nevertheless, some problems could be discussed as azotemia clearance insufficiency (5/34 cases) with this low blood and dialysate rate. This could be increased in hypercatabolic patients, but with some hypothermia or false normothermia. We did not observe either hemorrhagic problems or thrombocytopenia. In some high-risk patients, dialysis was performed without heparin, but with saline flush. In some other cases specially with multiple organ failure thrombosis of the lines appeared in spite of heparin control by anti-X factor activity. Acquired deficit of antithrombin III could be involved [4]. Other problems include transport of the patient (CT scan) or nurse acceptability which seems to be good with some organization.

References

1   Kron IL, Joob AW, van Meter C: Acute renal failure in the cardiovascular surgical patient. Ann Thorac Surg 1985;39:590–598.
2   Henrich W: Hemodynamic instability during hemodialysis. Kidney Int 1986;30:605–612.
3   Rasmussen H, Ibels L: Acute renal failure. Multivariate analysis of causes and risk factors. Am J Med 1982;73:211–218.
4   Bastien O, Saroul C, French P, Belleville J: Inefficacité de l'héparinothérapie par déficit acquis en antithrombine III lors d'hémodialyse continue. Presse Méd 1990;19:85.

Dr. O. Bastien, Département d'Anesthésie-Réanimation, Hôpital Cardiologique, B.P. Lyon Montchat, F–69394 Lyon Cedex 03 (France)

Sieberth HG, Mann H, Stummvoll HK (eds): Continuous Hemofiltration.
Contrib Nephrol. Basel, Karger, 1991, vol 93, pp 79–85

Slow Continuous Ultrafiltration: A Means of Unmasking Myocardial Functional Reserve in End-Stage Cardiac Disease

B. Canaud[a], *J.P. Cristol*[a], *K. Klouche*[b], *J.J. Béraud*[b], *G. Du Cailar*[c], *M. Ferrière*[d], *R. Grolleau*[d], *C. Mion*[a]

[a]Nephrology-Intensive Care Unit, [b]Metabolic-Intensive Care Unit, [c]Internal Medicine and [d]Cardiology, Lapeyronie University Hospital, Montpellier, France

End-stage cardiac disease (ESCD) may be readily described as a clinical syndrome characterized by severe congestive heart failure with diffuse edema, permanent dyspnea (grade IV, NYHA), low blood pressure, distended jugular vein, hepatomegaly and oliguric renal failure. Whatever the cause of myocardial damage (primary, ischemic, hypertensive, valvulopathy, toxic, metabolic) defect in myocardial contraction and inadequate cardiac output is a common result [1].

The morphologic and functional evaluation of left ventricular performance in ESCD usually demonstrates a dilated hypokinetic cardiomyopathy. A major cardiomegaly with pulmonary edema is observed on chest X-ray. A dilated left ventricle with reduced shortening index velocity is shown by echocardiography. A low ejection fraction is noted with radionuclide ventriculography [1].

ESCD is refractory to conventional medical treatment including rest, potent diuretics, various inotropic agents (cardioglycosides, dopamine, dobutamine) and/or vasodilatory agents [2–6]. ESCD results from a vicious circle linking the heart and the kidney in a mutual and progressive deterioration of function via neurohormoral changes and drug resistance as illustrated in figure 1 [7–10].

Slow continuous ultrafiltration (SCUF) or slow daily ultrafiltration (SDUF) appear the only procedure allowing the removal of large amounts of isotonic extracellular fluid (e.g. 150 mmol Na/l of ultrafiltrate removed) with good hemodynamic tolerance [11, 13]. Accordingly, we surmised that SCUF or SDUF would be an excellent method to break the vicious heart-kidney connection.

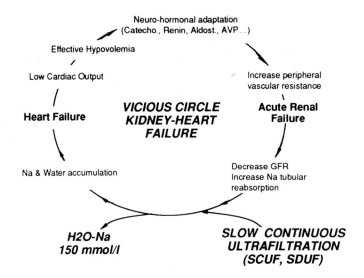

Fig. 1. Kidney-heart connection leading to mutual failure aggravation in congestive heart failure. SCUF impact-breaking site in this vicious circle.

Material and Methods

Patients. No particular selection criteria was used to contraindicate SCUF or SDUF in intractable ESCD patients. All patients referred to us with congestive heart failure (grade IV, NYHA) unresponsive to medical treatment including diuretics, inotropic and vasodilatory agents, were started on SCUF/SDUF. 35 patients (male: 27, female: 8; age: 62.6 ± 2.6 years) were included in this study protocol.

The following causes of cardiomyopathy were identified: ischemic heart disease 13, mixed hypertension and ischemia 12, valvular disease 5, nonobstructive cardiomyopathy 3, right heart disease secondary to chronic obstructive lung disease 1, toxic cardiomyopathy 1. Oliguric acute renal failure was present in all patients. In 27 patients, it was only functional, while in 8 patients chronic nephropathy with mild renal insufficiency existed prior to heart attack. A co-morbid state was identified in 9 patients: diabetes mellitus 5, chronic liver disease 1, polycystic kidney and liver disease 1, stabilized neoplasia 1, chronic obstructive lung disease 1.

Ultrafiltration Technique. Slow continuous ultrafiltration (SCUF) or slow daily ultrafiltration (SDUF) was performed via the venovenous circuit with a double and independent head pump monitor (BSM22, Hospal, Basel, Switzerland). The blood pump maintained a constant blood flow rate of 150–200 ml/min. The ultrafiltration pump ensured an adjustable ultrafiltration rate of 0.15–2 liters/h according to the cardiovascular stability of the patient (fig. 2).

Standard heparin (500–700 IU/h) or low-molecular-weight heparin (1,500–2,500 U/6 h) were used to prevent clotting of the extracorporeal circuit. Hemofilters (Biopal 2400S, AN69, flat sheet membranes, 1 m²; Filtral 12, AN69, capillary filter, 1.2 m²) were used ad libitum on SCUF and changed every day on SDUF. The major causes of filter changes were increased venous pressure above the alarm limit, reduced ultrafiltration rate or massive clotting of filter.

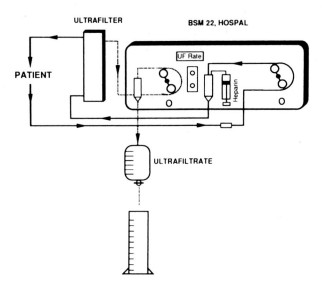

Fig. 2. Blood monitoring module used for SCUF/SDUF including a pump ultrafiltration-controlled system.

Vascular access was provided either by femoral catheters [19] or internal jugular silicone twin catheters [16].

Patient Follow-Up. Vital signs (blood pressure, heart rate, breath rate) and ultrafiltration rate were recorded hourly on a patient log chart. Clinical status, body weight, diuresis and fluid volume balance were evaluated daily. Biochemical analysis of blood and urine were done daily. Chest X-ray and ECG wer done every day during the first 7 days. Echocardiography and radionuclide ventriculography were performed when possible at the start and end of the treatment period.

Results

Treatment duration averaged 12 ± 2 days per patient including 3.3 ± 0.8 days (1–7 days) of SCUF/SDUF and 9 ± 2 days (4–21 days) of medical and drug therapy. Overall patient survival rate was 71.5% at the end of the first month, 40% at 12 and 34% at 24 months. Half-life survival rate could be estimated roughly to 10 months. In all cases, the cause of death was related to heart disease (sudden death). Multiple relapse episodes were noted in 7 patients requiring SCUF/SDUF for each new episode. One patient received a heart transplant after the second relapse episode but died 3 months later from acute ischemic arteriopathy.

Cumulative fluid volume removed by UF per patient was best estimated from body weight loss and averaged $19 \pm 3\%$ of the initial weight. Fluid volume removed by SCUF/SDUF was 4.3 ± 0.7 kg/day (2–10 kg/day) for

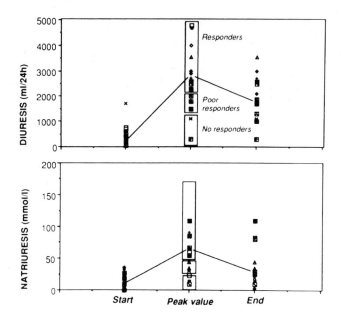

Fig. 3. Diuresis in ml/24 h (upper panel) and natriuresis in mmol/24 h (lower panel) in a group of congestive heart failure patients at initiation, peak response and end of SCUF/SDUF treatment period. As shown, 3 groups of patients (boxes) were identified according to their response to fluid volume depletion.

an average of 3 days. The body weight loss due to recovery of kidney function was 0.2 kg/day for 9 days permitting to reach the dry body weight. Diuresis and natriuresis increased after 2–3 days to reach a mean peak value of 2,500 ml/day and 70 (10–110 mmol/l) respectively, after the 3rd day. Large individual variations of diuresis and natriuresis were noted among the patients as presented in figure 3. Urea and creatinine concentration increased slightly after the acute volume depletion induced by SCUF, and return to within the normal range at the end of the follow-up period. A reduction in heart rate from 89 ± 4 to 81 ± 4 beats/min was observed, whereas mean arterial pressure did not change significantly (79 ± 2 vs. 81 ± 5 mm Hg). The cardiothoracic index was reduced from 0.65 ± 0.02 to 0.61 ± 0.02. Shortening index was increased from 0.18 ± 0.03 to 0.25 ± 0.02 (normal value 0.3). The ejection fraction measured in 5 patients improved from 0.30 to 0.40 (normal value 0.6). The plasma sodium concentration increased from 133 ± 1.2 (122–142 mmol/l) at the start to 136 ± 1.1 (130–145 mmol/l) at the end of the treatment period, while the plasma total protein concentration increased from 64 ± 1.5 (55–77 g/l) to 70 ± 2 (55–90 g/l).

Discussion

SCUF/SDUF is a simple and effective treatment modality for intractable congestive ESCD which permits, as hypothesized earlier, the vicious circle linking heart and renal failure to be broken [7, 9–15].

In spite of its apparent complexity due to the need of a pump-assisted and blood-monitoring module, SCUF was easily implemented and used routinely in our intensive care unit. SCUF via the venovenous-pump-driven system appears in many ways superior to the spontaneous arteriovenous approach which has been proposed [12–15].

Percutaneous catheterization of the deep vein was associated with a lower morbidity risk than arterial cannulation, especially in arteriopathic patients. The mechanically controlled ultrafiltration procedure ensured reliability and predictability in hemodynamically unstable patients. The pump-driven blood circuit maintained a regular and stable blood flow rate despite poor cardiac output and low pressure regimen. Moreover, ultrafiltration pump control allowed us to adjust the ultrafiltration rate to the hemodynamic conditions of the patients. A predominant depletion of extracellular fluid from the capacitance circuit by reducing the venous return flow rate relieves both the right ventricle work and the left ventricle preload without altering the effective blood volume [13].

Although no invasive hemodynamic investigations were performed in this study, indirect evidence suggests that SCUF acts in two ways. Firstly, ultrafiltration, the most powerful means to remove water and sodium in excess from body stores (150 mmol of sodium are taken out with each liter of fluid filtered) was able to restore a normal sodium pool in our patients. Accordingly, we roughly estimate that SCUF in our population removed 600 mmol/day within the first 3 days. Preload reduction obtained in this way relieves excessive myocardial stretching and permits the left ventricle to recover a sub-optimal functional level according to the Starling curve relationship. Secondly, SCUF appears to reduce the neurohormonal stimuli induced by heart failure which in turn lowers peripheral vascular resistance. This may be due to a reduced stretching of right atrial/ventricle sensors, but this remains purely speculative. However, this phenomenon is strongly suggested in our study by the brisk kidney functional changes noted during the course of SCUF. The paradoxical polyuria and the enhanced natriuresis observed during volume depletion in responder patients may therefore be viewed as a consequence of an increase in renal plasma flow with a subsequent enhanced glomerular filtration rate. Nevertheless, this interpretation remains purely speculative and further studies are required to elucidate this phenomenon.

The clinical results brought by this study also illustrate that SCUF/SDUF was a therapeutic means in desperate patients to unmask myocardial functional reserve. According to their response to SCUF three groups of patients were then identified. A first group, considered as 'responders' with rapid and prolonged remission after SCUF corresponds to patients with high cardiac functional reserve. A second group, considered as 'partial responders' with incomplete and temporary improvement and/or frequent relapse episodes corresponds to patients with poor cardiac functional reserve. A third group considered as 'no responders' with no cardiac or renal improvement corresponds to patients dying within the first month. Rapid reappearance of diuresis (polyuria) and significant natriuresis (> 50 mmol/l) appear to be a simple and reliable prognosis factors for further recovery.

We conclude that SCUF/SDUF should be considered on a short term basis, as a first-choice therapy for candidates to heart transplant, and on a long term basis, as comfort therapy in desperate terminal cases where heart transplant is contraindicated. On the other hand, SCUF might be viewed by the clinician as a 'negative' exercise test unmasking the cardiac functional reserve in each patient and giving a prognostic clue in severe congestive heart failure.

References

1   Braunwald E: Clinical manifestations of heart failure; in Braunwald E (ed): Heart Disease. Philadelphia, Saunders, 1988, pp 471–482.
2   Brater DC: Resistance to loop diuretics: Why it happens and what to do about it. Drugs 1985;30:425–477.
3   Lawson DH, Gary JMB, Henry DA, Tilstone WJ: Continuous infusion of furosemide in refractory oedema. Br Med J 1978;ii:476.
4   Crozier LG, Ikram H, Gomez HJ, Nicholls MG, Espiner EA, Warner NJ: Haemodynamic effects of atrial peptide infusion in heart failure. Lancet 1986;ii:1242–1245.
5   Gerlag PGG, Van Meijel JJM: High-dose furosemide in the treatment of refractory congestive heart failure. Arch Intern Med 1988;148:286–291.
6   Charbonnier B, Monpere B, Desveaux B, Cosnay P, Faucher JP, Brochier M: Traitement de l'insuffisance cardiaque chronique réfractaire par un inhibiteur de l'enzyme de conversion. Résultats à long terme. Ann Cardiol Angéiol 1984;33:233–237.
7   Francis GS, Goldsmith SR, Levine TB, Olivari MT, Cohn JN: The neuro-humoral axis in congestive heart failure. Ann Intern Med 1984;101:370–377.
8   Cody RJ, Atlas SA, Laragh JH, Kubo SH, Covit AB, Ryman KS, Shaknovich A, Podolfino K, Clark M, Camargo MJF, Scarborough RM, Lewicki JA: Atrial natriuretic factor in normal subjects and heart failure patients: plasma levels and renal, hormonal, and hemodynamic responses to peptide infusion. J Clin Invest 1986;78:1362–1374.
9   Mettauer B, Rouleau JL, Bichet D, Juneau C, Kortas C, Barjon JN, de Champlain J: Sodium and water excretion abnormalities in congestive heart failure: determinant factors and clinical implications. Ann Intern Med 1986;105:161–167.
10 Cody RJ, Covit AB, Schaer GL, Laragh JH, Sealey JE, Feldschuh J: Sodium and water balance in chronic congestive heart failure. J Clin Invest 1986;77:1441–1452.

11 Paganini EP: Slow continuous hemofiltration and slow continuous ultrafiltration. Trans ASAIO 1988;34:63–66.

12 Simpson JA, Rae AP, Simpson K, Gribben J, Boulton-Jones JM, Allison MEM, Hutton L: Ultrafiltration in the management of refractory congestive heart failure. Br Heart J 1986;55:344–347.

13 Rimondini A, Cipolla CM, Della Bella P, Grazi S, Sisillo E, Susini G, Guazzi MD: Hemofiltration as short-term treatment for refractory congestive heart failure. Am J Med 1987;83:43–48.

14 Canaud B, Cristol JP, Calvet B, Berthelemy C, Beraud JJ, Grolleau-Raoux R, Mion C: Traitement de l'insuffisance cardiaque réfractaire par ultrafiltration isolée; in Suc JM, Adler JL, Durand D, Ton That H (eds): Oedèmes Généralisés. Paris. Editions de Médecine Pratique, 1989, pp 195–205.

15 Canaud B, Cristol JP, Calvet B, Berthelemy C, Beraud JJ, Grolleau R, Garred LJ, Mion C: Significant improvement in survival rate of end-stage cardiac disease with slow continuous ultrafiltration. Blood Purif 1989;7:287–288.

Dr. Bernard Canaud, Division of Nephrology, Intensive Care Unit,
Lapeyronie University Hospital, 555, route de Ganges, F–34059 Montpellier (France)

Sieberth HG, Mann H, Stummvoll HK (eds): Continuous Hemofiltration.
Contrib Nephrol. Basel, Karger, 1991, vol 93, pp 86–89

Regulation of Acid-Base State with Hemofiltration in Circulatory Shock in Patients after Open Heart Surgery

F. I. Coraim, H. Haumer, W. Trubel, P. Simon

Clinic of Anesthesiology, University of Vienna, Austria

Maintenance of the acid-base balance in the extracellular space is accomplished through the mechanisms of systemic pH regulation:

$$pH = pK + \log HCO_3^- / CO_2.$$

The bicarbonate buffer plays a major role, since its components $HCO_3^- - CO_2$ are regulated very effectively through elimination. Therefore, mechanisms for the maintenance of pH homeostasis in the extracellular space must ensure a constant $HCO_3^- - CO_2$ relationship. Since CO_2 and HCO_3^- are continuously produced through metabolism, it is mandatory for the maintenance of pH homeostasis that it is eliminated at the same rate as it is produced. Classically, it is thought that systemic pH regulation is accomplished exclusively through the lungs and the kidney. In hemodynamically stable conditions with adequate alveolar ventilation, the CO_2 generated by $NaHCO_3^-$ can be eliminated by the lungs, and $NaHCO_3^-$ may therefore effectively neutralize excesses of H^+.

However, in cardiogenic shock during ischemia coronary blood flow is reduced and anaerobic myocardial metabolism results in the production of H^+, CO_2 and lactate. CO_2 is the predominant determinant of muscle pH. Extracellular HCO_3^- has only a minor effect on intracellular pH. Partial 'respiratory compensation' of extracellular metabolic acidosis readily prevents intracellular acidosis; however, increases in extracellular HCO_3^- fail to correct intracellular acidosis. The bicarbonate buffering of anaerobically generated lactate may explain increases in intramyocardial CO_2. Increases in myocardial CO_2 are associated with reduced myocardial contractility [1, 2]. Venous blood-gas data – in contrast to arterial – reflect with greater accuracy the actual acid-base state of the tissues during cardiogenic shock. Neither CO_2 generating or CO_2 consuming buffer agents improve the acid-base status [2–4]. They probably additionally have adverse effects on tissue oxygenation and myocardial function [5, 6]. In cardiogenic shock, hypoxia leads to metabolic breakdown, resulting in metabolic lactic acidosis, increased proteolysis, and elevated ammonia levels. These changes are associated with decreases of myocardial performance. The aim of this study was to evaluate the presence of amino acid imbalance and of increased lactate and ammonia levels in the circulation of patients with shock, and to assess the beneficial effect of hemofiltration on acid base regulation.

Methods

Two groups of patients (group I: in cardiogenic shock, n = 28; group II: control, n = 23) were evaluated. Group I underwent hemofiltration.

Results

The bicarbonate level in group I was 16.4 ± 3.9 compared with group II 25 ± 2.4 mmol/l which was insignificantly low. The ammonia level in group I was 61 ± 37 mmol/l, but reached 24 ± 6.4 mmol/l in the control group. The lactate value in the shock group (group I) increased to 18.5 ± 9 mmol/l and compared with the control group was significantly enhanced ($p < 0.01$). The relative glutamine level in group I decreased significantly to $13.4 \pm 4\%$. This demonstrates the disturbance of ammonia binding. It was possible to decrease the values by hemofiltration, thereby normalizing the acid base status.

Discussion

Amino acid metabolism in the liver produces not only ammonia but also CO_2 and bicarbonate. The elimination of HCO_3^- and ammonia produced in the proteolysis is accomplished in the liver through urea synthesis. However, in cardiogenic shock hypoxia leads to metabolic breakdown, which results in metabolic lactic acidosis and increased proteolysis. An accelerated breakdown of proteins and amino acids in high amounts produced increased ammonia concentration. Ammonia must be removed from the circulation since it is neurotoxic. The acidosis promotes accelerated amino acid degradation. In particular, glutamine and aspargin synthesis are inhibited which results in decreased renal excretion of ammonia and proton elimination through the glutamic acid synthesis. This aggravates the clinical condition of the patients. Circulatory failure is by far the most common cause of lactic acidosis in intensive care medicine. The magnitude of the lactatemia reflects the severity of the circulatory failure and it is directly related to mortality [2]. An equimolar quantity of H^+ is produced with the lactate and titrates in tissue and blood bicarbonate; the bicarbonate is restored when the lactate is converted to electroneutral products such as glucose, glycogen or CO_2, and water. This conversion takes place mainly in the liver (40–70%) but also in kidney, heart and under some circumstances in resting skeletal muscle. The energy production is much more critically affected in the liver and the kidney during shock which probably also reflects the higher metabolic activity and energy needs of these organs. Both these organs are normally of importance for the clearance of lactate formed in other tissues, but in shock states when tissue hypoxia ensues also in the liver and kidney this lactate-metabolizing ability may be lost. The liver and the kidney may then themselves turn into lactate-producing organs, a situation that signals a severe deterioration of metabolic control. Lactate acidosis also appears to have direct negative effects on myocardial function [3, 4]. This effect appears to be most pronounced when the acidosis is due to hypoxia, as myocardial contractile function is depressed more by the combination of hypoxia and lactic acidosis than by either process alone [5]. Since tissue oxgyen delivery is critically dependent upon cardiac output in hypoxic states and cardiopulmonary arrest, the negative inotropic effect of lactic acidosis assumes a critically important role in determining the clinical outcome in these situations [2]. Unfortunately, the therapy of lactic acidosis has been problematic because of the fact that the most commonly employed therapeutic agent, sodium bicarbonate, has not been consistently demonstrated either to elevate arterial pH or to lower the blood lactate concentration, and it probably has adverse effects on tissue oxygenation and myocardial function as well. Bicarbonate buffering of the anaerobically generated lactate may explain increases in intramyocardial CO_2 [6]. Adverse effects of hypercapnia involve primarily the cardiovascular and central nervous systems, including increased adrenergic activity. Increases in myocardial CO_2, are associated with reduced myocardial contractility. Progressive hypercarbic acidosis favors the competition of H^+ ions with calcium ions for binding to troponin and cross-bridging between actin and myosin is therefore inhibited. The dysfunction of the sarcoplasmic reticulum with decreases in both calcium uptake and ATPase activity may be responsible for the ultimate breakdown in the myocardial excitation-contraction coupling system. Indeed, recent data from Korestunne et al. [5] demonstrated fourfold increases in free intracellular calcium during ventricular fibrillation which would further account for decreases in myocardial contractility and prolonged postresuscitation contractile dysfunction, known as stunned myocardium [5]. Further side effects of $NaHCO_3^-$ include, among others, increases in plasma osmolality, left shifts of the oxyhemoglobin dissociation curve and hypernatremia, all of which are potentially deleterious. THAM was an efficient buffer agent with consumed CO_2 but exerted arterial vasodilator effects which of themselves adversely affected outcome [6]. Carbicarb failed to decrease coronary vein CO_2 or to mitigate intramyocardial acidosis or to improve resuscitability. In such a situation, hemofiltration is an excellent method to treat the metabolic disturbance and to eliminate the humeral component of cardiogenic shock followed by highly improved hemodynamics and tissue oxygenation.

References

1 Arieff AI, Gertz EW, Park R et al: Lactic acidosis and the cardiovascular system in the dog. Clin Sci 1983;64:573–580.

2 Bersin RN, Arieff AI: Improved hemodynamic function during hypoxia with carbicard a new agent for the management of acidosis. Circulation 1988;77:277.

3 Cooper DJ, Worthley LIG: Adverse haemodynamic effects of sodium bicarbonate in metabolic acidosis. Intens Care Med 1987;13.

4 Ichihara K, Haga N, Yasushi A: Is ischemia-induced pH decrease of dog myocardium respiratory or metabolic acidosis. Am J Physiol 1984;246:H652–657.

5 Korestune Y, Marban G: Cell calcium in the pathophysiology of ventricular fibrillation and in the pathogenesis of postarrhythmic contractile function. Circulation 1989;80:369–379.

6 von Planta M, Weil MH, Gazmuri RJ et al: Myocardial acidosis associated with CO_2 production during cardiac arrest and resuscitation. Circulation 1989;80:684–692.

F.I. Coraim, MD, Lustkandlgasse 18/5, A–1090 Vienna (Austria)

Sieberth HG, Mann H, Stummvoll HK (eds): Continuous Hemofiltration.
Contrib Nephrol. Basel, Karger, 1991, vol 93, pp 90–93

Regulatory Effect of Neurotransmitter by Hemofiltration in Cardiogenic Shock Patients after Open Heart Surgery

F.I. Coraim, Alyson Owen, W. Trubel, H. Kassal, K. Widhalm

Department of Anesthesiology and Intensive Care, University of Vienna, Austria

In the postoperative care after open heart surgery cerebral dysfunction still remains a complex clinicopathological problem in patients with cardiogenic shock. Up to now in these cases the classic concept of brain dysfunction has focussed an alteration of ammonia level ratio of BCAA/AAA, and GABA concentration in the blood [4]. However, the ultimate role for BCAA in the treatment of hepatic encephalopathy (HE) is uncertain [1]. Also little is known about hypoxia-induced general cell dysfunction leading to an imbalance of excitatory and inhibitory neurotransmitters. The aim of this study was to correlate the occurrence of excitatory and inhibitory amino acids (glutamate, aspartate and glycine, respectively) and the ammonia levels in blood to neurological abnormalities (Glasgow coma scale) in cardiogenic shock after coronary artery bypass grafting (CABG). Based on these data the benefit of hemofiltration on neurological symptoms in cardiogenic shock was investigated.

Patients and Methods

Fifty-two patients who had undergone CABG were entered in this study. Twenty-eight patients were in cardiogenic shock after the operation (16 male, 12 female, age range 18–67 years) with a HE grade III (20) and IV (8). Twenty-three of these shock patients received hemofiltration (HF). Twenty-three patients after CABG without cardiogenic shock (16 male, 7 female, age range 35–67 years) served as the control group. Cardiogenic shock was defined by decreased cardiac index, SVI, left ventricular stroke work index and critical reduction of SVO_2 ($<60\%$). All shock patients were under mechanical ventilation and showed typical hemodynamic instability despite administration of catecholamines at high dosage. All patients were examined for neurological symptoms, which were graded according to the Glasgow coma scale (table 2) and the stage of HE (table 1). The clinical grading of HE was performed immediately before initiation of HF or 12–20 h postoperatively. In all groups repeated measurements of serum lactate, ammonia, amino acids and blood gas analysis were performed.

Table 1. Hepatic encephalopathy stage (modified by Conn [5])

Stage	Shock group (n = 28)		Control group (n = 23)
	before HF (n = 23)	without HF (n = 5)	
I	0	0	20
II	2	0	3
III	13	2	0
IV	8	3	0
Survivors	17	0	23
Nonsurvivors	6	5	0

Table 2. Degree of coma (according to the Glasgow scale)

Score	Shock group (n = 28)		Control group (n = 23)
	before HF (n = 28)	after HF (n = 23)	
15–20	0	17	20
10–15	19	0	3
<10	9	6	0

Results

On admission to the ICU, 2 patients were in a HE stage II, 15 in HE stage III and 11 in HE stage IV (table 1). Seventeen patients (all after hemofiltration) progressed to coma stage I and survived. The remaining 6 patients from the hemofiltrated group showed a temporary improvement accompanied by a decrease of laboratory parameters within 3–7 days of HF treatment. However, subsquently their hemodynamic state deteriorated and all of these 6 patients died. In all 5 patients not receiving hemofiltration treatment the neurological status further deteriorated rapidly due to cerebral edema (verified by CT scan) and all of them died within 12 h. In the control group no changes in clinical and laboratory parameters were observed.

Discussion

The basic problem in cardiogenic shock is an insufficient nutritive blood flow to tissue, i.e. a critically disturbed supply to demand of oxygen resulting in tissue hypoxia and cellular anaerobiosis. Moreover, in the early

Table 3. Amino acid ratio (%) and ammonia serum level (mmol/l)

	Shock group (n = 28)		Control group (n = 23)
	before HF (n = 28)	after HF (n = 23)	
Glutamate	2.9 ± 2	2.0 ± 1.7*	1.1 ± 0.9*
Aspartate	6.3 ± 8	0.4 ± 0.3*	0.21 ± 0.03*
Glycine	14.8 ± 8	8.9 ± 2.7*	7.4 ± 1.5*
Ammonia	61 ± 37	22 ± 4*	23 ± 6*

* p < 0.01, Student's t test.

phase of shock there is a pronounced neurohumeral activation in an initial increase of metabolic drive. The blood levels of glucose, amino acids, free fatty acids, glycerol as well as lactate are thus increased to cover the cellular metabolic response in shock. Experimental studies indicate that the liver may in fact be a very critical target organ in shock. Energy failure in the liver according to its decreased ischemic tolerance at the time of shock treatment will reduce the overall clearing capacity for amino acids and other metabolites and may thereby critically affect survival. Therefore, the liver is unable to remove these amino acids from the circulating blood and because of the increased release of amino acids, a characteristic amino acid pattern is found in the blood of experimental animals and of patients with hepatic insufficiency and encephalopathy (table 3). The mechanism of the mental disorder in cardiogenic shock is, at least to some degree, similar to that of hepatic encephalopathy. The transition of neurotransmitters to neurotoxin by limited cellular energy were shown in cerebral neurons in the shock state. Large increase in level of excitatory amino acid neurotransmitters were found in brain regions during ischemia and recirculation, and was suggested to be one of the causal factors of ischemic brain damage. Ammonia continues to be considered as an important neurotoxin and may act synergistically with other toxic substances [2, 3].

Several studies confirmed the development of cerebral edema in 75–80% of patients in grade III–IV encephalopathy and is one of the major causes of death. In an animal model an unspecific increase of permeability of the blood-brain barrier could be demonstrated in acute hepatic encephalopathy. Increased permeability facilitates the development of cerebral edema and the uptake of neurotoxins. The increase in permeability itself may be caused by ammonia and other neurotoxins [4].

It has been suggested that hemofiltration, by minimizing systemic osmotic gradients, would be a better approach than hemodialysis and would diminish both, the incidence and severity of cerebral edema. It therefore is concluded, that hemofiltration is an excellent method to eliminate such neurotoxic substances and to normalize the amino acid concentrations in the brain leading to an improved neurological condition.

References

1 Alexander WF, Spindel E, Harty RF et al: The usefulness of branches chain amino acids in patients with acute or chronic hepatic encephalopathy. Am J Gastroenterol 1989, pp. 91–96.

2 Loscher W, Kretz FJ, Tung LC et al: Reduction of highly elevated plasma levels of gamma-aminobutyric acid does not reverse hepatic coma. Hepatogastroenterology 1989, pp. 504–505.

3 Mizock BA, Sabelli HC, Dubin A et al: Septic encephalopathy. Evidence for altered phenylalanine metabolism and comparison with hepatic encephalopathy. Arch Intern Med 1990;150(2):443–449.

4 Naylor CD, Rourke O, Detsky AS et al: Perenterale nutrition with branched-chain amino acids in hepatic encephalopathy. A meta-analysis. Gastroenterology 1989;4:1033–1042.

5 Conn HO, Lieberthal MM: The Hepatic coma Syndromes and laktulose. Williams and Wiltkins Co Baltimore 1979, pp 4–8.

F.I. Coraim, MD, Lustkandlgasse 18/5; A–1090 Vienna (Austria)

Sieberth HG, Mann H, Stummvoll HK (eds): Continuous Hemofiltration.
Contrib Nephrol. Basel, Karger, 1991, vol 93, pp 94–97

Continuous Arteriovenous Hemofiltration in the Adult Respiratory Distress Syndrome

A Randomized Trial

Frank Cosentino, Emil Paganini, John Lockrem, James Stoller, Herbert Wiedemann

The Cleveland Clinic Foundation, Cleveland, Ohio, USA

Continuous arteriovenous hemofiltration (CAVH) and slow continuous ultrafiltration have emerged as effective modalities in the management of acute renal failure (ARF). More recently, this form of therapy has received attention for nonrenal applications such as the adult respiratory distress syndrome (ARDS) and multiorgan failure [1–3].

To assess the potential benefits of CAVH in the management of ARDS, we conducted a randomized controlled trial to evaluate the effects of CAVH on pulmonary and hemodynamic parameters as well as survival of patients with ARDS. Patients in the control group received standard supportive therapy for ARDS; subjects that were randomized to the treatment group underwent standard supportive treatment plus CAVH.

Patients and Methods

At study entry all patients was assigned an APACHE II score [4]. Patients with APACHE II scores less than 20 were randomized to control or treatment groups. Subjects with scores of 20 or greater were randomized in a similar fashion. Because of small patient numbers, results were analyzed comparing all control patients (n = 6) to all treatment patients (n = 9).

Criteria for the diagnosis of ARDS was based on the clinical criteria put forth by Pepe et al. [5]. These criteria along with the associated clinical setting for our patients are depicted in table 1. Patients were excluded from study entry if there was evidence of cardiogenic pulmonary edema (pulmonary wedge pressure > 18 mm Hg), evidence of pneumonia (purulent sputum with positive cultures) or serious central nervous system disorders (head trauma or raised intracranial pressure).

CAVH was performed utilizing femoral arterial and venous access, a polyamide hemofilter and standard bicarbonate replacement solution. The ultrafiltration rate was 12 ± 0.8 liters/day. CAVH was performed for 5–7 days. If control patients developed ARF, requiring dialysis, they underwent standard hemodialysis utilizing a polyacrylonitrile membrane. Two control patients and one patient in the treatment group required dialytic support for ARF.

Table 1. Criteria for clinical diagnosis of ARDS

Pulmonary parameters
1. $PaO_2 < 75$ mm Hg with $FIO_2 > 0.50$
2. Diffuse pulmonary infiltrate on chest X-radiography
3. Pulmonary capillary wedge pressure < 18 mm Hg

Clinical setting
1. Sepsis (n = 10)
2. Pancreatitis (n = 3)
3. Multiple transfusions during emergency resuscitation (n = 1)
4. Unknown (n = 1)

Table 2. Hemodynamic parameters (mean ± SEM)

	Study entry	Study conclusion	p value
Control group (n = 6)			
MAP, mm Hg	78.8 ± 7.97	86.9 ± 5.08	n.s.
Weight, kg	86.8 ± 10.70	96.0 ± 9.31	n.s.
CI, l/min/m²	5.03 ± 0.52	5.71 ± 0.33	n.s.
PCWP, mm Hg	14.8 ± 1.20	16.0 ± 2.49	n.s.
CAVH group (n = 9)			
MAP, mm Hg	90.58 ± 7.45	78.39 ± 3.00	n.s.
Weight, kg	79.98 ± 4.43	79.79 ± 5.48	n.s.
CI, l/min/m²	4.57 ± 0.21	4.81 ± 0.49	n.s.
PCWP, mm Hg	15.33 ± 0.60	15.63 ± 1.08	n.s.

MAP = Mean arterial pressure; CI = cardiac index; PCWP = pulmonary capillary wedge pressure.

Results

Outcome events included hemodynamic data and gas exchange parameters analyzed for differences at study entry and at the conclusion of the study period which was 6.1 ± 0.4 days. Table 2 shows the hemodynamic parameters for both groups at study entry and conclusion. Over the study period there was no significant change for either group. Both groups experienced essentially even fluid balance as depicted by no significant changes in body weight or pulmonary wedge pressures.

Table 3 shows the gas exchange parameters for control and treatment subjects at the beginning and conclusion of the study period. Although no significant changes occurred in the treatment group, the control group demonstrated reduced FIO_2 requirements (p = 0.04) and enhanced

Table 3. Gas exchange parameters (mean ± SEM)

	Study entry	Study conclusion	p value
Control group (n = 6)			
FIO$_2$	0.65 ± 0.09	0.47 ± 0.03	0.04
PaO$_2$, mm Hg	78.6 ± 13.01	94.4 ± 15.66	n.s.
PEEP, cm H$_2$O	12.60 ± 1.25	13.40 ± 1.89	n.s.
DO$_2$	744.20 ± 129.03	906.20 ± 85.89	n.s.
VO$_2$	186.22 ± 15.76	246.62 ± 14.08	0.02
CAVH group (n = 9)			
FIO$_2$	0.53 ± 0.05	0.55 ± 0.06	n.s.
PaO$_2$, mm Hg	70.89 ± 3.50	77.22 ± 9.05	n.s.
PEEP, cm H$_2$O	13.44 ± 1.51	12.11 ± 1.52	n.s.
DO$_2$	661.43 ± 60.22	788.17 ± 116.93	n.s.
VO$_2$	163.96 ± 17.77	159.20 ± 14.07	n.s.

PEEP = Positive end-expiratory pressure; DO$_2$ = oxygen delivery; VO$_2$ = oxygen consumption.

oxygen consumption (p = 0.02). Other parameters (PaO$_2$/FIO$_2$ and oxygen delivery) demonstrated nonsignificant trends of improvement for the control group.

In spite of the lack of improvement in hemodynamic and gas exchange parameters in the treatment group, the results showed a nonsignificant trend of enhanced survival for the subjects receiving CAVH. Survival for the treatment group was 56% (5/9) compared to 17% (1/6) for the control group (p = 0.29).

Discussion
Interpretation of results is difficult since the trend of enhanced survival in the treatment group is at odds with the improved gas exchange parameters in the control group. Small patient numbers may account for this apparent discrepancy. The role of CAVH in ARDS remains unclear. Some studies have found a benefit [1, 3, 6] while others have not [7, 8]. Certainly additional research is needed.

References
1   Barzilay E, Kessler D, Lesmes C, Lev A, Weksler N, Berlot G: Sequential plasmafilter-dialysis with slow continuous hemofiltration: Additional treatment for sepsis-induced AOSF patients. J Crit Care 1988;3:163–166.
2   Gotloib L, Barzilay E, Shustak A, Lev A: Sequential hemofiltration in nonoliguric high capillary permeability pulmonary edema of severe sepsis: Preliminary report. Crit Care Med 1984;12:997–1000.

3 Gotloib L, Barzilay E, Shustak A, Wais Z, Jaichenko J, Lev A: Hemofiltration in septic ARDS: The artificial kidney as an artificial lung. Resuscitation 1986;13:123–132.
4 Knaus WA, Draper EA, Wagner DP, Zimmerman JE: APACHE II: A severity of disease classification system. Crit Care Med 1985;13:818–829.
5 Pepe PE, Potkin RT, Reus DH: Clinical predictors of the adult respiratory distress syndrome. Am J Surg 1982;144:124–130.
6 Romano E, Gullo G, Kette F: Pulmonary gas exchange in critically ill patients during continuous arteriovenous hemofiltration (CAVH). Int Symp on Continuous Arteriovenous Hemofiltration. Milan, Wichtig, 1986, pp 139–145.
7 Koller W: Continuous arteriovenous hemofiltration in ICU patients with pulmonary disorders. Int Symp on Continuous Arteriovenous Hemofiltration. Milan, Wichtig, 1986, pp 331–346.
8 Sznajder JI, Zucker AR, Wood LDH, Long GR: The effects of plasmapheresis and hemofiltration on canine acid aspiration pulmonary edema. Am Rev Respir Dis 1986;134:222–228.

Dr. F. Cosentino, Department of Hypertension and Nephrology,
The Cleveland Clinic Foundation, 9500 Euclid Ave., Cleveland,
OH 44195 (USA)

Sieberth HG, Mann H, Stummvoll HK (eds): Continuous Hemofiltration.
Contrib Nephrol. Basel, Karger, 1991, vol 93, pp 98–104

Acute Renal Failure following Cardiac Surgery: Pre- and Perioperative Clinical Features

H. Schmitt[a], *J. Riehl*[a], *A. Boseila*[c], *A. Kreis*[b], *A. Pütz-Stork*[a],
H.B. Lo[c], *H. Lambertz*[b], *B.J. Messmer*[c], *H.G. Sieberth*[a]

Departments of Internal Medicine [a]II and [b]I, and [c]Thoracic and Cardiovascular
Surgery, Technical University of Aachen, FRG

Acute renal failure is a serious complication of cardiac surgery. With the increasing performance of heart operations – in particular coronary artery bypass surgery – the problem of postoperative renal failure has become more important during recent years.

Several studies dealing with acute renal failure after cardiac surgery have been published from 1962 to 1988 [1–16]; a survey is shown in table 1. The data are difficult to compare because of marked differences in definitions and selection criteria. Altogether 380 patients were evaluated; the incidence of severe renal failure was similar in all investigators ranging from 0.8 to 5.6% with 2.7% on average. The majority reported a fairly high mortality rate of 65–92% [1, 3–9,11, 13–16]; only three groups found substantially better results [2, 10, 12].

In our hospital, acute renal failure requiring renal replacement therapy occurred in 1.7% among nearly 5,000 patients undergoing open heart surgery from 1985 to 1989. The incidence was higher in valve replacement as compared to bypass operation (2.6 vs. 0.9%); with a combined surgical procedure it even increased to 4.5% (table 2). The mortality rate corresponded well with the data known from the literature (table 2).

A critical circulation caused by different factors is reported to play an important role in the pathogenesis of acute postoperative renal dysfunction [16]. In order to define risk factors we analyzed a series of clinical variables in a large group of patients with serious acute renal failure following cardiac surgery.

Patients

In total we studied 81 patients – 51 male, 30 female – with a mean age of 61.7 years. Table 3 describes the types of surgical procedures. Valve replacement and bypass operation were equally distributed. Fourteen percent of all operations were performed as an emergency intervention, either for unstable angina pectoris or advanced heart failure or acute endocarditis.

Table 1. Acute renal failure following cardiac surgery: incidence and mortality rate

	Incidence, % (n)	Mortality, %
Doberneck et al., 1962 [1]	3.0 (30/1,000)	87
Yeh et al., 1964 [2]	5.6 (10/180)	10
Porter et al., 1967 [3]	2.9 (6/209)	68
Johansson et al., 1967 [4]	3.1 (13/423)	92
Porter and Starr, 1969 [5]	1.3 (12/911)	67
Yeboah et al., 1972 [6]	4.7 (20/428)	70
Abel et al., 1976 [7]	3.6 (18/500)	89
Bhat et al., 1976 [8]	4.3 (21/490)	67
Krian, 1976 [9]	5.3 (157/2,945)	72
Mc Leish et al., 1977 [10]	1.6 (25/1,542)	28
Hilberman et al., 1979 [11]	2.5 (5/204)	65
Gailiunas et al., 1980 [12]	1.5 (11/752)	27
Heikkinen et al., 1985 [13]	0.9 (15/1,686)	67
Koning et al., 1985 [14]	1.9 (27/1,403)	–
Morgan et al., 1988 [15]	0.8 (10/1,600)	–
Average	2.7 (380/14,273)	61

Table 2. Acute renal failure following cardiac surgery: incidence and mortality rate (present series) (total number of operations: 4995; Jan. 1985–July 1989)

	Incidence, %	Mortality, %
All cases (n = 81)	1.7	68
Aortocoronary bypass graft (ACBG)	0.9	75
Valve replacement (VR)	2.6	57
ACBG + VR	4.5	73

Results and Discussion

Preoperative impairment of renal function was a surprising but frequent finding. Although it was mild in most patients, there were some with creatinine levels exceeding 300 µmol/l (table 4). Only 39% exhibited completely normal renal function.

Pre-existing heart failure was also frequently observed. According to the NYHA criteria, one third of our patients had to be classified as advanced congestive heart failure (table 5). This was confirmed by routinely obtained chest X-ray; signs of right-sided, left-sided or biventricular heart failure were demonstrable in a total of 51%. Global left ventricular performance was calculated during echocardiography by measuring ejection fraction, fractional shortening and end-diastolic diameter. The degree of left ventricular dysfunction was moderate in 33% and severe in 23%

Table 3. Acute renal failure following cardiac surgery: types of surgical procedures

Surgical procedure	%	n
Aortocoronary bypass graft (ACBG)		28
Single ACBG	4	
Double ACBG	32	
Triple ACBG	32	
Four or more grafts	32	
Valve replacement (VR)		28
Aortic VR	39	
Mitral VR	39	
Double VR	22	
Combination of ACBG and VR		22
Miscellaneous		3

Table 4. Acute renal failure following cardiac surgery: preoperative renal function

Renal function	%
Normal renal function	39
Mild renal failure (creatinine 100–150 μmol/l)	46
Moderate renal failure (creatinine 151–300 μmol/l)	10
Severe renal failure (creatinine >300 μmol/l)	5

Table 5. Acute renal failure following cardiac surgery: preoperative classification of heart failure according to the NYHA criteria

Classification	%
NYHA I	2
NYHA II	18
NYHA III	47
NYHA IV	33

(table 6). Furthermore, enlargement of the right heart cavities was observed in more than 40% indicating pre-existing pulmonary hypertension.

The main preoperative electrocardiographic features were ischemia plus hypertrophy and myocardial infarction in the past with 38 and 32%

Table 6. Acute renal failure following cardiac surgery: preoperative echocardiographic features

Echocardiographic feature	%
Left ventricular function	
Normal	44
Moderate dysfunction	33
Severe dysfunction	23
Right ventricular size	
Normal	58
Enlarged	42

Table 7. Acute renal failure following cardiac surgery: preoperative rhythm disturbances

Rhythm disturbance	%
Sinus rhythm	69
Atrial fibrillation	31
Ventricular ectopic beats (Lown classification)	
Normal findings	58
⩽ Lown III	26
⩾ Lown IVa	16

respectively. With regard to rhythm disturbances, our data are summarized in table 7. Atrial fibrillation was present in nearly one third of our patients whereas frequent and complex ventricular premature beats could only be recognized in a minor percentage.

With cardiac catheterization including selective angiography of the coronary arteries the most common pathological finding was a triple vessel disease (25%) followed by a double and a single vessel disease (16% and 11% respectively). A main stem stenosis of the left coronary artery was observed in 9%. In another 39% of our patients we could not reveal any significant obstructive lesions within the main branches of the coronary arteries. The values of some important hemodynamic variables are depicted in table 8. Mean cardiac index was low, but still within the normal limits. The distribution within our group, however, shows a diminished cardiac index in 32%. The corresponding and simultaneously recorded left ventricular end-diastolic pressure was elevated in 70%. Moreover, an increase in mean pulmonary artery pressure was found in 60% with an average value amounting to 28 mm Hg. This hemodynamic pattern indicates a significant

Table 8. Acute renal failure following cardiac surgery: preoperative cardiac catheterization data

Cardiac catheterization data	%
Left ventricular end-diastolic pressure 17 ± 10 mm Hg ($\bar{x} \pm$ SD)	
Normal	30
Elevated	70
Cardiac index 2.7 ± 0.7 l/min $\cdot$ m^2 ($\bar{x} \pm$ SD)	
Decreased	32
Normal	66
Increased	2
Mean pulmonary artery pressure 28 ± 14 mm Hg ($\bar{x} \pm$ SD)	
Normal	40
Elevated	60

impairment of left ventricular function as well as an additional increase in pulmonary vascular resistance.

Some intraoperative and early postoperative clinical data are presented in table 9. The relatively long duration of the operation in total, and of cardiopulmonary bypass and aortic cross-clamping in particular, can be interpreted as a general indicator of major intraoperative problems. Corresponding to this finding severe systemic hypotension with temporary systolic blood pressure below 80 mm Hg was observed in more than 70% of our patients. This unstable hemodynamic condition was furthermore complicated by recurrent ventricular fibrillation. Despite additional application of catecholamines, treatment with the intra-aortic balloon pump was required in 45%. Intraoperative bleeding complications with consecutive systemic hypotension are one of the most important causes of postoperative renal failure. This is reflected by the large number of patients who received substitution of blood components during cardiac surgery.

Various factors may contribute to a critical circulation during and after cardiac surgery thus leading to acute renal failure. A prolonged period of cardiopulmonary bypass is generally considered to be one of the major risk factors in the development of postoperative renal dysfunction [1, 3, 6–9, 11, 13, 14]. The duration of aortic cross-clamping, the total duration of the operation and pre-existing renal damage also closely correlated with the incidence of acute renal failure [3, 6, 7, 9]. The deleterious effect of systemic hypotension on renal perfusion is well known [1, 8, 13, 14]. The significance of several other parameters – such as age, type of operation, NYHA classification, ventricular function, and

Table 9. Acute renal failure following cardiac surgery: intraoperative data

Total duration of the operation, min	271 ± 118
Cardiopulmonary bypass time, min	155 ± 85
Aortic cross-clamping time, min	75 ± 29
Lowest systolic intraoperative blood pressure, %	
>120 mm Hg	1
$101 - 120$ mm Hg	4
$81 - 100$ mm Hg	24
$60 - 80$ mm Hg	53
<60 mm Hg	18
Intra- and early postoperative complications, %	
No complications	8
Severe systemic hypotension	67
Recurrent ventricular fibrillation	3
Hypotension + ventricular fibrillation	22
Intraoperative administration of catecholamines, %	
No catecholamines	5
Epinephrine	8
Epinephrine + dopamine	87
Use of cardiac assist devices (aortic counterpulsation), %	
Intra-aortic balloon pump (IABP)	45
No IABP support	55
Intraoperative substitution of blood components, %	
Packed red blood cells or whole blood	
No transfusion	10
1–5 units	78
6–10 units	9
>10 units	3
Fresh frozen plasma	
No substitution	71
1–3 units	24
>3 units	5

left ventricular end-diastolic pressure – remains controversial [1, 3, 6–9, 11, 13, 14]. Some of these previously published potential risk factors, however, have only been studied in small numbers of patients. In our group of 81 patients we frequently found a preoperative impairment of renal function and signs of left- and right-sided heart failure shown by different methods of examination. The significance and the predictive value of these striking features, however, has to be confirmed by further studies considering a valid control group.

With regard to the poor prognosis of acute renal failure following cardiac surgery, Abel et al. [7] pointed out in 1976: 'Therapy of this postoperative complication, therefore, appears to be better directed toward its prevention rather than treatment once established'.

References

1   Doberneck RC, Reiser MP, Lillehei CW: Acute renal failure after open-heart surgery utilizing extracorporeal circulation and total body perfusion. Analysis of one thousand patients. J Thorac Cardiovasc Surg 1962;43:441–452.

2   Yeh TJ, Brackney EL, Hall DP, Ellison RG: Renal complications of open heart surgery: predisposing factors, prevention, and management. J Thorac Cardiovasc Surg 1964;47:79–97.

3   Porter GA, Kloster FE, Herr RJ, Starr A, Griswold HE, Kimsey J: Renal complications associated with valve replacement surgery. J Thorac Cardiovasc Surg 1967;53:145–152.

4   Johansson L, Lundberg S, Söderlund S: Renal complications following heart surgery with extracorporeal circulation. Scand J Thorac Cardiovasc Surg 1967;1:52–56.

5   Porter GA, Starr A: Management of postoperative renal failure following cardiovascular surgery. Surgery 1969;65:390–398.

6   Yeboah ED, Petrie A, Pead JL: Acute renal failure and open heart surgery. Br Med J 1972;i:415–418.

7   Abel RM, Buckley MJ, Austen WG, Barnett GO, Beck CH, Fischer JE: Etiology, incidence, and prognosis of renal failure following cardiac operations. Results of a prospective analysis of 500 consecutive patients. J Thorac Cardiovasc Surg 1976;71:323–333.

8   Bhat JG, Gluck MC, Lowenstein J, Baldwin DS: Renal failure after open heart surgery. Ann Intern Med 1976;84:677–682.

9   Krian A: Incidence, prevention, and treatment of acute renal failure following cardiopulmonary bypass. Int Anaesthesiol Clin 1976;14:87–101.

10 Mc Leish KR, Luft FC, Kleit SA: Factors affecting prognosis in acute renal failure following cardiac operations. Surg Gynecol Obstet 1977;145:28–32.

11 Hilberman M, Myers BD, Carrie BJ, Derby G, Jamison RL, Stinson EB: Acute renal failure following cardiac surgery. J Thorac Cardiovasc Surg 1979;77:880–888.

12 Gailiunas P, Chawla R, Lazarus JM, Cohn L, Sanders J, Merrill JP: Acute renal failure following cardiac operations. J Thorac Cardiovasc Surg 1980;79:241–243.

13 Heikkinen L, Harjula A, Merikallio E: Acute renal failure related to open-heart surgery. Ann Chir Gynaecol 1985;74:203–209.

14 Koning HM, Koning AJ, Leusink JA: Serious acute renal failure following open heart surgery. Thorac Cardiovasc Surg 1985;33:283–287.

15 Morgan JM, Morgan C, Evans TW: Clinical experience of pumped arteriovenous haemofiltration in the management of patients in oliguric renal failure following cardiothoracic surgery. Int J Cardiol 1988;21:259–267.

16 Kron IL, Joob AW, van Meter C: Acute renal failure in the cardiovascular surgical patient. Ann Thorac Surg 1985;39:590–598.

Dr. H. Schmitt, Medizinische Klinik II, Klinikum der RWTH, Pauwelsstrasse 30, D-W-5100 Aachen (FRG)

Sieberth HG, Mann H, Stummvoll HK (eds): Continuous Hemofiltration.
Contrib Nephrol. Basel, Karger, 1991, vol 93, pp 105–109

Influence of Continuous Hemofiltration on Hemodynamics and Pulmonary Function in Porcine Endotoxic Shock

B. Stein, E. Pfenninger, A. Grünert, A. Deller

Klinik für Anästhesiologie, Universitätsklinik Ulm, FRG

The combination of acute renal failure and acute respiratory distress syndrome remains an important expression of multiple organ failure, caused by sepsis and septic shock [1–3].

The early initiation of renal replacement therapy such as continuous hemofiltration is an accepted therapeutic approach in this situation [2, 3]. However, the interference of this procedure with pulmonary dysfunction in sepsis is not well understood [4, 5]. Clinical and pathophysiologic considerations assume two possible interactions: (1) an influence on the interstitial pulmonary edema and the hydrostatic pressures in the pulmonary circulation by positive or negative balancing [4], and (2) the alteration of lung damage during sepsis by the convective transport of mediator substances through the hemofilter [5–7].

In order to evaluate the importance of the second mechanism, we studied the effect of a 'zero-balanced hemofiltration' with a high ultrafiltration rate on endotoxin-induced changes in lung mechanics, extravascular lung water and pulmonary circulation in an endotoxic shock model, and compared it to the spontaneous course.

Methods

In 20 domestic pigs of either sex (28–30 kg body weight), under general anesthesia with intubation and mechanical ventilation, graded endotoxinemia was evoked until doubling of the mean pulmonary pressure was reached [time 1 (PAP_{max})]. The necessary dose of endotoxin was then halfed and the animals randomly assigned either to receive zero-balanced venovenous hemofiltration with a simultaneous ultrafiltration and replacement rate of 600 ml/h (10 animals) or to observe the spontaneous course (10 animals) under a constant infusion of endotoxin for 4 h (time 2–5). There was no additional therapy with fluids or catecholamines. Priming dose, priming time and endotoxin infusion rate were similar in both proups. Zero-balanced hemofiltration was achieved by controlling the prescribed ultrafiltration and substitution rate of 600 ml/h by means of two infusion pumps.

Extravascular lung water and central blood volume were determined simultaneously by the thermo-dye double-indicator technique using a 5-french fiberoptic probe in the aorta descendens (PV 2024 FO-TD, Cold System, Pulsion, Munich, FRG). Central blood volume represents the distribution volume of indigocyanin green between the site of injection at the right atrium (10 ml aqua ad inj. at 1–1.5 °C, Indigocyanin green 0.25%) and signal perception in the aorta. Cardiac output, mean pulmonary artery pressure (PAP) and pulmonary capillary wedge pressure (PCWP) were determined by a Swan Ganz catheter. The respiratory pressure-volume loop (P/V loop) was analyzed as a slow dynamic compliance with inflation and deflation of 600 ml over 20 s with a supersyringe, using a lung function measurement unit (Pulmostar SM, Fenyves & Gut, Basel, Switzerland).

Statistical analysis was performed by analysis of variance (ANOVA), t test for independent paired data from both groups and Mann-Whitney U test for nonnormally distributed data. $p < 0.05$ was regarded as significant.

Results

The survival rate of hemofiltrated animals at time 4 and at the end of the experiment (time 5) was not statistically significantly different compared to the spontaneous course. The time course of central blood volume and cardiac output revealed a constant decrease in both parameters in the spontaneous course. This trend of central blood volume was not altered by hemofiltration, whereas the time course of cardiac output in the hemofiltrated animals showed a distinct difference in the ANOVA procedure and a significant higher mean value at one point (time 4) of measurement.

Parameters of pulmonary circulation as mean PAP, PCWP and pulmonary vascular resistance (PVR) showed a biphasic course, with an initial maximal increase during endotoxin priming and a second slower increase toward the end of the experiment (fig. 1). Continuous hemofiltration lowered significantly PAP at time 2 and 3, PCWP at time 2 and 4, as demonstrated in figure 1, and PVR at time 3. Extravascular lung water showed a slight but insignificant increase in both groups without differences between the two groups. Analysis of the P/V loops, obtained during the course of the experiment, included the slope of the P/V loop, representing the total compliance of the respiratory system, the hysteresis area and the slope of the inspiratory and expiratory limb of the P/V loop. A progressive increase in hysteresis area was evident during endotoxinemia and the spontaneous course, whereas this increase was prevented by hemofiltration with significant lower mean values at time 3 and 4 (fig. 2).

Analysis of the compliance of inflation and deflation showed significant differences with higher mean values for the hemofiltrated animals at time 3 and 4.

Discussion

The design of this investigation did not allow fluid resuscitation with the consequence that a hypovolemic and hypodynamic endotoxic shock was produced in both groups, represented by the fall of cardiac output and central blood volume. The modification of lung mechanics and pulmonary

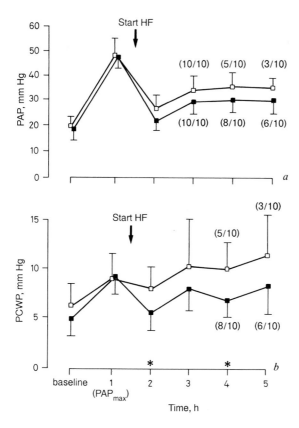

Fig. 1. Mean PAP (a) and PCW (b) during the stages of the experiment. □ = Endotoxin-treated group, spontaneous course (n = 10); ■ = endotoxin-treated and hemofiltrated group (n = 10). Statistical significance (spontaneous vs. hemofiltrated group): *p < 0.005. HF = Hemofiltration.

hemodynamics in this porcine endotoxic shock model by zero-balanced hemofiltration cannot be explained by an impact on the intravascular volume status. This is excluded by the methodical approach of the zero-balancing technique as well as by the time course of central blood volume. Therefore, our results must be distinguished from the well-known effects on hemodynamics and pulmonary edema by negative balancing [4].

The design of this investigation and data from other clinical and experimental studies support the hypothesis that the filtration of small- and medium-sized mediator substances, such as thromboxane A_2 [5] and interleukins [7], could play a role in the explanation of these findings.

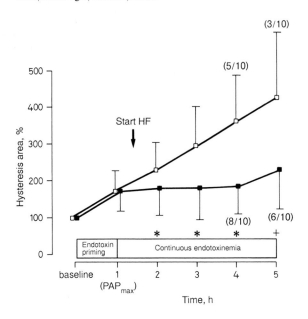

Fig. 2. Hysteresis area as percent of baseline value during the stages of the experiment. □ = Endotoxin-treated group, spontaneous course (n = 10); ■ = endotoxin-treated and hemofiltrated group (n = 10). Statistical significance (spontaneous vs. hemofiltrated group): *p < 0.005. HF = Hemofiltration.

Even respecting the cautious interpretation of the experimental data, obtained with a small number of animals studied, the trend of the parameters of lung mechanics and pulmonary circulation toward baseline values may be interpreted as a decrease in entoxin-induced pulmonary damage by continuous hemofiltration. In accordance with clinical observations [2–5], these data support the early initiation of hemofiltration in the therapeutic plan of sepsis and septic shock, when a combination of impaired renal and pulmonary function is evident.

References

1   Sweet SJ, Glenney CU, Fitzgibbons JP, Friedmann P, Teres D: Synergistic effect of acute renal failure and respiratory failure in the surgical intensive care unit.

2   Simpson K, Allison M: Acute renal failure-continuous ultrafiltration and bicarbonate haemodialysis (CUPID). Intensive Care World 1988;5:83–84.

3   Wendon J, Smithies M, Sheppard M, Bullen K, Tinker J, Bihari D: Continuous high volume venous-venous haemofiltration in acute renal failure. Intensive Care Med 1989;15:358–363.

4   Wilkowski A, Goeckenjan G: Auswirkungen des Flüssigkeitsentzugs auf pulmonale Verlaufsparameter und Prognose des akuten Lungenversagens. Intensivmedizin 1988;25:10–16.
5   Gotloib L, Barzilay E, Shustak A, Wais Z, Jaichenko J, Lev A: Hemofiltration in septic ARDS: The artificial kidney as an artificial endocrine lung. Resuscitation 1986;13:123–132.
6   Staubach KH, Rau HG, Kooistra A, Schardey HM, Hohlbach G, Schildberg FW: Can hemofiltration increase survival time in acute endotoxinemia? A porcine shock model (abstract). Second Vienna Shock Forum, Vienna, May 1988, p 69.
7   Gross D, Dahan JB, Landau EH, Krausz MM: Effect of leukotriene inhibitor LY-171883 on the pulmonary response to *Escherichia coli* endotoxinemia. Crit Care Med 1990;18:190–197.

Dr. Bernhard Stein, 31, rue du Téméraire, F–54000 Nancy (France)

Pharmacokinetics

Sieberth HG, Mann H, Stummvoll HK (eds): Continuous Hemofiltration.
Contrib Nephrol. Basel, Karger, 1991, vol 93, pp 110–116

Drug Removal during Continuous Hemofiltration or Hemodialysis

Thomas A. Golper

Kidney Disease Program, University of Louisville, Ky., USA

Hemofiltration

Sieving Coefficient. Solute removal during hemofiltration (HF) is convective. The sieving cofficient, S, is the solute concentration in the ultrafiltrate/solute conc. in the retentate. S is the mathematical expression of the solute's ability to convectively permeate a membrane. An S of 1 states that the solute freely passes while an S of O describes complete rejection. Colton et al. [1] have shown that a reasonable approximation is:

$$S = \frac{UF}{\frac{A+V}{2}} = \frac{2\,UF}{A+V},$$

where A, V, and UF represent the arterial, venous and ultrafiltrate concentrations, respectively. Golper et al. [2] have further shown that under CAVH conditions, $S = UF/A$ which elinimates the need for a venous sample. Strictly speaking, when determining S, A and V should represent the plasma water conc. of the solute. Since plasma water makes up about 95% of plasma, this distinction can be ignored for clinical purposes.

Under conditions of CAVH or CVVH, S will generally be constant [3, 4]. With very high transmembrane pressures S may decrease for large molecules [5, 6]. Presumably, retarding protein layers (protein concentration polarization) or protein-membrane interactions decrease sieving. There is no evidence that this occurs during CAVH. Furthermore, solute sieving is independent of blood flow [4, 5]. During HF clearance is the product of S times the ultrafiltration rate (UFR). Since S is constant, clearance is linearly related to UFR. Thus, the most important way to describe drug handling in CAVH is to determine its S.

Kronfol and co-workers [7–9] have demonstrated that in the absence of confounding proteins, there are drug membrane interactions during

CAVH. S's for several drugs through PAN and polyamide membranes were significantly different from those through polysulfone. Drug charge could affect either convective or diffusive transport, depending on the nature of the drug-membrane charge interaction. We found that cationic gentamicin *in saline* had an S through polysulfone of only 0.94 [4]. Lysaght [10] has shown that even the sodium cation has an S less than unity. The introduction of a negative charge on macromolecules can decrease sieving during HF [11]. However, small anions such as chloride and bicarbonate have S's greater than unity [12, 13], thought to be secondary to the Gibbs-Donnan effect of circulating proteins.

Rumpf et al. [14] first suspected that drugs bound to dialysis membranes. Kraft and Lode [15] noted gentamicin binding to RP-6, while Kronfol et al. [16] described tobramycin and amikacin binding to AN69S. We recently confirmed this [17]. When aminoglycosides bind to membranes, S is very low for the first few minutes after exposure, but as the binding sites saturate, S rises. A Biospal filter binds 10–20 mg of tobramycin [16].

Binding to nonultrafilterable plasma proteins will play a dominant role in determining a drug's convective transport. Protein-bound drug will not be filtered. Many factors affect drug-protein binding including pH, molar concentration of drug and protein, bilirubin, uremic inhibitors, heparin, free fatty acids, and the presence of displacing drugs [18–26]. The unbound drug is the pharmacologically active fraction. If there is displacement, the pharmacologic effect, metabolism, and removal will be enhanced. To point out the complexity of the issue, free fatty acids may displace cefamandole, but may enhance the binding of other cephalosporins like cephalothin or cefoxitin [24]. We have shown that free fatty acids increase the S of phenytoin [4].

Table 1 displays the S and unbound fraction (alpha) of drugs whose S has been determined either from my experience or the literature. These data are plotted in figure 1 showing the significant correlation between S and alpha.

The role of molecular size (weight and steric hindrance) on membrane transport has been extensively studied [1, 5, 6, 27, 28]. For most drugs in clinical use, molecular size will not be an issue for removal during HF. The membrane molecular weight cutoffs exceed the molecular weight of the drugs.

Drug Removal during HF. Inulin readily traverses polysulfone hemofilter membranes [5, 27, 29]. Since virtually all therapeutic agents have a molecular weight less than that of inulin, one can reasonable assume that these drugs will permeate these membranes limited mostly by the extent of

Table 1. Drug-sieving coefficients (S) in CAVH compared to unbound fraction (a)

Antibiotics			Other		
drug	S	a	drug	S	a
Amikacin	0.9	0.9	Bromide	1.0	1.0
Amphotericin	0.3	0.1	Chlorodiazepoxide	0.05	0.05
Ampicillin	0.7	0.8	Cisplatin	0.1	0.1
Cefoperazone	0.3	0.1	Clofibrate	0.06	0.04
Cefotaxime	0.5	0.6	Cyclosporine	0.6	0.1
Cefoxitin	0.3	0.3	Diathybarbital	1.0	0.9
Ceftazidime	0.9	0.9	Diazepam	0.02	0.02
Ceftriaxone	0.8	0.1	Digoxin	0.9	0.8
Cephapirin	1.5	0.6	Famotidine	0.7	0.8
Cilastin	0.8	0.6	Glibenclamide	0.6	0.01
Clindamycin	1.0	0.4	Glutethimide	0.02	0.5
Doxycycline	0.4	0.2	Lidocaine	0.2	0.4
Erythromycin	0.4	0.3	Metamizole	0.4	0.4
Gentamicin	0.8	0.9	NAP	0.9	0.9
Imipenem	1.2	0.9	Nitrazepam	0.08	0.1
Metronidazole	0.8	0.8	Nomifensin	0.7	0.4
Mezlocillin	0.7	0.7	Oxazepam	0.1	0.1
Nafcillin	0.5	0.2	Phenobarb	0.8	0.6
Netilmicin	0.9	0.9	Phenytoin	0.4	0.4
Oxacillin	0.02	0.05	Procainamide	0.9	0.9
Penicillin	0.7	0.5	Pyrithyldione	0.4	–
Streptomycin	0.3	0.6	Theophylline	0.9	0.5
Sulfamethoxazole	0.9	0.6			
Tobramycin	0.8	0.9			
Vancomycin	0.8	0.9			

$r = 0.67$; $p < 0.001$.

their protein binding. Protein-binding data are available, usually from studies of healthy people [30]. Slight discrepancies may arise when comparing those data to critically ill patients.

One can measure the removal of drug during HF by multiplying the UF drug conc. by the UFR. Since (arterial) plasma levels are usually required for clinical management, one could calculate the UF concentration from the arterial concentration (A) by the formula:

UF = A × alpha

where the protein binding is *assumed* to be normal [30]. The following summarizes the technique to determine drug removal from CAVH: (1) Deter-

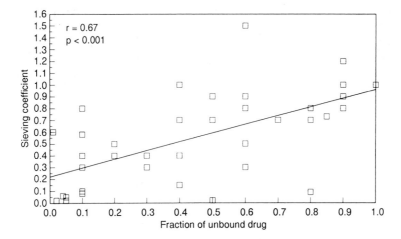

Fig. 1. Drug-sieving coefficients (S) during either high flux hemofiltration, CAVH or simulated CAVH. S is plotted versus the fraction of drug unbound to plasma proteins, calculated from reference 30. By linear regression analysis, there is a significant correlation. n = 45 drugs.

mine steady-state arterial concentration (A). (2) Determine fraction *not* bound to protein (alpha) [30]. (3) Determine UFR. (4) Amount removed = A × unbound fraction × UFR.

The arterial sample should represent a steady-state level. The ideal time to obtain it is halfway between maintenance doses after at least 3 half-lives. $T^1/_2$ data are also available [30].

Hemodialysis

During CAVHD drug removal occurs mostly by diffusion. Protein binding still plays a role in that unbound drug is more diffusable than bound drug. As molecular volume (weight + ionic drag) increases, there is decreased diffusivity through hemodialysis (HD) membrane pores, approximated by a negative linear relationship between the log of dialysance and the log of molecular weight [31]. A drug approaching a molecular weight of 500 daltons will be marginally dialyzed through conventional membranes whereas vancomycin at 1,400 daltons is appreciably dialyzed through more open membranes like those employed in CAVHD [32]. As molecular weight increases, dialyzer clearance becomes less dependent on blood and dialysate flow rates and more dependent on the convective component [33].

Solute losses during combined convection and diffusion are less than the sum of each transport process individually [34]. Convection impairs diffusion in hemodiafiltration (HDF) and in CAVHD to a lesser extent [33]. The presence of convectively derived solute in the dialysate decreases the concentration gradient, the driving force for diffusion. This can be overcome by increasing dialysate flow rate. During CAVHD a 500-dalton molecule has a clearance less than that of urea [33, 35]. Nonetheless, during HDF a similar molecule was cleared at a rate twice that of conventional HD [36].

During HDF as transmembrane pressure increases, protein concentration polarization occurs and protein bound drugs are brought into proximity to other protein-bound drug molecules, other protein molecules, the membrane, and dialysate. Several of these potential interactions could result in drug displacement from its binding site. Thus, the transport of this drug across the membrane may be further enhanced by both the steep concentration gradient (diffusion) and the proximity induced displacing interactions caused by the convective component. Thus, HDF may clear drugs greater than either HD or HF.

Supplemental Doses

Drug levels are a utilizable tool when the desired level is known. Both loading and maintenance doses can be determined. The presently observed level (present level) is subtracted from the level one wishes to achieve (desired level) leaving the *difference level* all in the same units. The difference level times the volume of distribution times the body weight in kilograms will give the amount of drug needed to boost the present level to the desired level.

For loading doses, the present level is zero and the difference level is the desired level. For maintenance doses, the trough level is the present level. This method is useful for administering any drug whose level is available and whose V_d is known. It is especially applicable to the setting of CAVH when the amount of drug removed by the renal replacement therapy is not clearly known and the clinician has only drug levels to assess the pharmacologic status of the patient. V_d data are readily available [30].

References

1   Colton CK, Henderson LW, Ford CA, Lysaght MJ: Kinetics of hemodiafiltration. I. In vitro transport characteristics of a hollow fiber blood ultrafilter. J Lab Clin Med 1975;85:355–371.
2   Golper TA, Wedel SK, Kaplan AA, Saad AM, et al: Drug removal during CAVH: Theory and clinical observations. Intern J Artif Organs 1985;8:307–312.
3   Ronco C, Brendolan A, Borin D, Bragantini L, et al: Permeability characteristics of polysulfonic membranes in CAVH; in Sieberth HG, Mann H (eds):Continuous Arteriovenous Hemofiltration (CAVH). Basel, Karger, 1985, pp 59–63.

4 Golper TA, Saad AM: Gentamicin and phenytoin in vitro sieving characteristics through polysulfone hemofilters: Effect of flow rate, drug concentration and solvent systems. Kidney Int 1986;30:937–943.

5 Frigon RP, Leypoldt JK, Alford MF, Uyeji S, et al: Hemofilter solute sieving is not governed by dynamically polarized protein. Trans ASAIO 1984;30:486–490.

6 Klein E, Holland FF, Eberle K: Rejection of solutes by hemofiltration membranes. ASAIO J 1978;1:15–23.

7 Kronfol NO, Lau AH, Colon-Rivera J, Libertin CL: Effect of CAVH membrane types on drug sieving coefficients and clearances. Trans ASAIO 1986;32:85–87.

8 Lau A, Kronfol N, Jaber N, Libertin C: Determinants of drug removal by continuous arteriovenous hemofiltration. Drug Intell Clin Pharm 1986;20:467.

9 Kronfol N, Lau A, Jaber N, Libertin C: Effect of membrane properties on drug clearances by CAVH. Abstr National Kidney Found Ann Meet, 1986, p A10.

10 Lysaght MJ: An experimental model for the ultrafiltration of sodium ion from blood or plasma. Blood Purif 1983;1:25–30.

11 Leypoldt JK, Frigon RP, Henderson LW: Macromolecular charge affects hemofilter solute sieving. Trans ASAIO 1986;32:384–387.

12 Kaplan AA, Longnecker RE, Rolkert VW: Continuous arteriovenous hemofiltration - a report of 6 months' experience. Ann Intern Med 1984;100:358–367.

13 Paganini EP, Flague J, Whitman G, Nakamoto S: Amino acid balance in patients with oliguric renal failure undergoing slow continuous ultrafiltration (SCUF). Trans ASAIO 1982;28:615–620.

14 Rumpf KW, Rieger J, Ansorg R, Dohl B, Scheler F: Binding of antibiotics by dialysis membranes and its clinical relevance. Proc EDTA 1977;14:677–688.

15 Kraft D, Lode H: Elimination of ampicillin and gentamicin by hemofiltration. Klin Wochenschr 1979;57:195–6.

16 Kronfol NO, Lau AH, Barakat MM: Aminoglycoside binding to polyacrylonitrile hemofilter membranes during continuous hemofiltration. Trans ASAIO 1987;33:300–303.

17 Cigarran-Guldris S, Brier ME, Golper TA: Tobramycin clearance during simulated continuous arteriovenous hemodialysis; in Sieberth HG, Mann H, Stummvoll HK (eds): Continuous Hemofiltration. Contrib Nephrol. Basel, Karger, 1991, vol 93, pp 120–123.

18 Reidenbery MM, Affrime M: Influence of disease on binding of drugs to plasma proteins. Ann NY Acad Sci 1973;226:115–126.

19 Dayton PG, Israili ZH, Perel JM: Influence of binding on drug metabolism and distribution. Ann NY Acad Sci 1973;226:172–194.

20 Anton AH: Increasing activity of sulfonamides with displacing agents. Ann NY Acad Sci 1973;226:273–292.

21 Reidenberg MM: The binding of drugs to plasma proteins and the interpretation of measurements of plasma concentration of drugs in patients with poor renal function. Am J Med 1977;62:466–470.

22 Tillement JP, Lhoste F, Findicelli TF: Diseases and drug protein binding. Clin Pharmacokinet 1978;3:144–154.

23 McNamara PJ, Lalka D, Gibaldi M: Endogenous accumulation products and serum protein binding in uremia. J Lab Clin Med 1981;98:730–740.

24 Suh B, Craig WA, England AC, Elliott RL: Effect of free fatty acids on protein binding of antimicrobial agents. J Infect Dis 1981;143:609–610.

25 Gulyassy PF, Depner TA: Impaired binding of drugs and endogenous ligands in renal disease. Am J Kidney Dis 1983;2:578–601.

26   Keller F, Wilms H, Schultze G, Offerman G, et al: Effect of plasma protein binding, volume of distribution and molecular weight on the fraction of drugs eliminated by hemodialysis. Clin Nephrol 1983;19:201–205.

27   Leypoldt JK, Frigon RP, Henderson LW: Dextran sieving coefficients of hemofilter membranes. Trans ASAIO 1983;29:678–683.

28   Rockel A, Gilge U, Liewald A, Heidland A: Elimination of low molecular weight proteins during hemofiltration. Artif Organs 1982;6:307–317.

29   Dodd NJ, O' Donovan RM, Bennett-Jones DN, Rylance PB, et al: Arteriovenous hemofiltration: A recent advance in the management of renal failure. Br Med J 1983;287:1008–1010.

30   Bennett WM, Aronoff GR, Golper TA, Morrison G, Singer I: Drug prescribing in renal failure: Dosing guidelines for adults. Ann Intern Med 1987.

31   Henderson LW: Hemodialysis: Rationale and physical principles; in Brenner RM, Rector FC (eds): The Kidney, ed 1. Philadelphia, Saunders, 1976, pp 1643–1671.

32   DeBock V, Verbeelen D, Maes V, Sennesael J: Pharmacokinetics of vancomycin in patients undergoing haemodialysis and haemofiltration. Nephrol Dial Transplant 1989;4:635–639.

33   Golper TA, Cigarran-Guldris S, Jenkins RD, Brier ME: The role of convection during simulated continuous arteriovenous hemodialysis; in Sieberth HG, Mann H, Stummvoll HK (eds): Continuous Hemofiltration. Contrib Nephrol. Basel, Karger, 1991, vol 93, pp 146–148.

34   Sprenger KGB, Stephen H, Kratz W, Huber K, Franz HE: Optimizing of hemodiafiltration with modern membranes? Contrib Nephrol. Basel, Karger, 1985, vol 46, pp 43–60.

35   Geronemus R, Schneider N, Miale A, Kotler J: Middle molecule clearance in CAVHD. Kidney Int 1987;31:232.

36   Basile C, DiMaggio A, Curino E, Scatizzi A: Pharmacokinetics of netilmicin in hypertonic hemodiafiltration and standard hemodialysis. Clin Nephrol 1985;24:305–309.

Thomas A. Golper, MD, Kidney Disease Program, 500 S. Floyd Street, Louisville, KY 40292 (USA)

Sieberth HG, Mann H, Stummvoll HK (eds): Continuous Hemofiltration.
Contrib Nephrol. Basel, Karger, 1991, vol 93, pp 117–119

Clearance Studies in Patients with Acute Renal Failure Treated by Continuous Arteriovenous Haemodialysis

Stephen P. Davies, Wolfgang J. Kox, Edwina A. Brown

Charing Cross and Westminster Medical School, London, UK

Continuous arteriovenous haemodialysis (CAVHD) is now an established technique for the treatment of acute renal failure (ARF) which is well tolerated by critically ill and unstable patients. By combining diffusive and convective transport, clearances of small-molecular-weight solutes are higher than with standard continuous arteriovenous haemofiltration [1]. This means that CAVHD can be used as a sole form of renal replacement therapy in even the most catabolic of patients with ARF without the need for supplemental haemodialysis [2]. However, the majority of drugs used in clinical practice are also of relatively low molecular weight. If the clearances of these are similarly high during CAVHD, the doses administered might need to be increased. On theoretical grounds, the removal of larger molecules should be primarily by convection and, therefore, losses of these substances are unlikely to be high as large ultrafiltration volumes are generally neither desired nor attained during CAVHD.

The aims of the present study were the following: (1) to measure the clearances of a range of small-molecular-weight solutes in patients with ARF treated by CAVHD; (2) to measure the clearances of some of the drugs commonly used in the treatment of these patients, and (3) to measure the clearances of β_2-microglobulin (β_2M) as a higher molecular-weight substance of 11,800.

Materials and Methods

CAVHD was performed using Hospal AN69S 0.43-m^2 polyacrylonitrile filters (Hospal AN69S, SCU/CAVH, Hospal, UK) and standard 1.5% dextrose peritoneal dialysis fluid (Fresenius CAPD/DPCA 2). The dialysate was run through the filter at either 1 or 2 litres/h, with the rate being controlled by an infusion pump. In all patients, vascular access was via Scribner arm or leg shunts and the unpumped blood circuit was routinely anticoagulated with heparin, 10 IU/kg/h. In those considered to be at high risk of haemorrhage, prostacycline, 2–5 ng/kg/min, was used either alone or with a reduced heparin dose.

Table 1. CAVHD solute clearances (mean ± SEM) at dialysate flow rates (Q_d) of 1 and 2 litres/h

Substance	Clearance, ml/min		p value
	Q_d 1	Q_d 2	
Urea	22.02 ± 0.46	33.46 ± 0.81	<0.001
Creatinine	20.15 ± 0.48	29.43 ± 0.80	<0.001
Phosphate	20.68 ± 0.70	28.26 ± 1.12	<0.001
Urate	16.49 ± 0.54	22.21 ± 0.75	<0.001
β_2M	6.58 ± 0.65	6.62 ± 0.78	n.s.
Cefuroxime	13.97 ± 2.34	16.22 ± 3.35	n.s.
Ceftazidime	13.11 ± 1.15	15.24 ± 1.47	<0.01
Ciprofloxacin	16.31 ± 1.89	19.93 ± 1.11	n.s.
Vancomycin	11.70 ± 1.88	15.58 ± 2.07	<0.01
Tobramycin	11.10 ± 1.89	14.85 ± 1.17	n.s.
Gentamicin	20.51 ± 2.12	25.94 ± 2.72	<0.05
Digoxin	10.04 ± 1.23	10.96 ± 0.93	n.s.
Doxycycline	6.99 ± 0.55	12.11 ± 1.69	n.s.

Blood specimens were collected from the venous and arterial blood lines, and samples of spent dialysate/ultrafiltrate were taken from the exit point of the filter in order to calculate clearances at dialysate flow rates of both 1 and 2 litres/h. Whenever the dialysate flow rate was changed, an interval of at least 20 min was allowed before specimens were collected to ensure equilibration under the new conditions. Ultrafiltration rates were calculated from 30-min collection volumes. In patients studied on more than one occasion, repeat studies were performed at least 24 h apart using different filters.

Dialysate clearances were calculated using a standard formula [3]. All results are expressed as mean ± SEM. Differences in the clearances at the two dialysate flow rates were analysed using the paired t test.

Clearances of the small-molecular-weight solutes urea, creatinine, phosphate and urate (all n = 40) were measured, together with the clearances of cefuroxime (n = 6), ceftazidime (n = 5), ciprofloxacin (n = 10), vancomycin (n = 10), tobramycin (n = 7), gentamicin (n = 4), digoxin (n = 6) and doxycycline (n = 2) in patients receiving these drugs. Clearances of β_2M were measured in 16 patients.

Results and Discussion

The results are summarised in table 1. Clearances of small solutes including most drugs were higher at a dialysate flow rate of 2 litres/h than at 1 litre/h. This failed to reach statistical significance for many of the drugs, however, because of the small number of studies involved. Increasing the dialysate flow rate did not significantly increase clearance of β_2M. Instead, this correlated closely with the ultrafiltration rate (r = 0.75, p < 0.001; fig. 1).

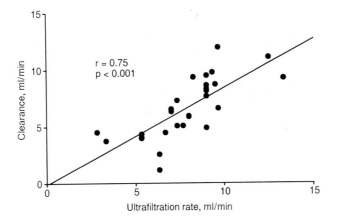

Fig. 1. β_2M clearance versus ultrafiltration rate.

We have confirmed that CAVHD is highly effective at removing small-molecular-weight solutes including a number of antibiotics. In contrast, we have demonstrated that, as expected on theoretical grounds, the clearance of larger molecules such as β_2M depends primarily on convection. Losses of such molecules are therefore unlikely to be of significance when using this system of renal replacement therapy which does not depend primarily for its effectiveness on achieving high ultrafiltration rates.

References

1   Sigler MH, Teehan BP: Solute transport in continuous hemodialysis: A new treatment for acute renal failure. Kidney Int 1987;32:562–571.
2   Stevens PE, Riley B, Davies SP, Gower PE, Brown EA, Koxw W: Continuous arteriovenous haemodialysis in critically ill patients. Lancet 1988;150–152.
3   Henderson LW: Biophysics of ultrafiltration and hemofiltration; in Drukker W, Parsons FM, Maher J (eds); Replacement of Renal Function by Dialysis. Boston, Nijhoff, 1983, pp 242–264.

Dr. S.P. Davies, Research Fellow, Department of Medicine, Charing Cross Hospital, Fulham Palace Road, London W6 8RF (UK)

Sieberth HG, Mann H, Stummvoll HK (eds): Continuous Hemofiltration.
Contrib Nephrol. Basel, Karger, 1991, vol 93, pp 120–123

Tobramycin Clearance during Simulated Continuous Arteriovenous Hemodialysis

Secundino Cigarran-Guldris, Michael E. Brier, Thomas A. Golper

University of Louisville, Ky., USA

Aminoglycoside clearance has been described in hemodialysis [1], hemofiltration [2], hemodiafiltration [3] and during continuous arteriovenous hemofiltration [4–6], but not during continuous arteriovenous hemodialysis (CAVHD). Because tobramycin is commonly prescribed and has useful pharmacological characteristics, it should serve as a prototypic drug for evaluation of clearance during CAVHD. It was studied as part of an investigation into the principles of solute clearance during CAVHD under conditions of maximum ultrafiltration rate (UFR) and dialysate flow rate (Q_d). Data regarding the clearances of urea and inulin are described in the companion paper in this volume [7].

Materials and Methods

Heparinized human plasma, obtained during therapeutic apheresis, was dialyzed free of glucose, azide-treated to retard bacterial growth and supplemented with urea (60 daltons) to 70 mg/dl, tobramycin (500 daltons) (Eli Lilly, Indianapolis, Ind., USA) to 8 mg/l and inulin (5,200 daltons) to 100 mg/dl. At 37 °C it was pumped single-pass through either Renaflo HF500 or HF250 (Renal Systems, Minneapolis, Minn., USA), Amicon D20 or D30 (Danver, Mass., USA) or Biospal (Hospal, Meyzieu, France) hemofilters. The HF500, D30 and Biospal are comparably large surface area filters while the HF250 and D30 are comparably sized smaller filters. Glucose-free standard hemodialysate from concentrate (Renal Systems) was pumped countercurrently. Plasma flow was 60 ml/min throughout. Q_d entering the hemofilter was either 15, 30 or 60 ml/min. Dialysate outflow rate was adjusted to generate UFRs of 0, 5, 10 or 20 ml/min. Each filter was studied in triplicate and each combination of flows in duplicate for each filter.

Tobramycin was assayed on Abbott TDX® (fluorescence polarization immunoassay).

Data were analyzed by analysis of variance. Statistical significance was achieved if $p < 0.05$.

Results and Discussion

Figure 1 displays the tobramycin clearance in the large filters at the extremes of Q_d for all UFRs. Although for each filter a greater clearance is noted for Q_d of 60 ml/min, the difference is not great. Figure 2 is a similar

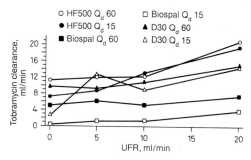

Fig. 1. Tobramycin clearances in comparably sized large filters (HF500, D30 and Biospal) at the extremes of Q_d and dependence on UFR. Each data point is the mean of 6 observations.

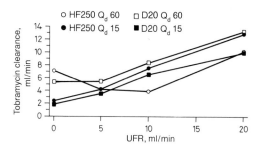

Fig. 2. Tobramycin clearances in comparably sized small filters (HF250 and D20) at the extremes of Q_d and dependence on UFR. Each data point is the mean of 6 observations.

display for the two smaller filters. The D20 demonstrated a greater tobramycin clearance at Q_d for 60 ml/min than at Q_d 15 ml/min, but the HF250 did not. For all the filters combined, there was a significant contribution to clearance by increasing the Q_d. As Q_d increased from 15 to 60 ml/min, tobramycin clearance increased by 22%. Thus, the results are reproducible but not great in magnitude. Of all the filters studied, the Biospal, known as an excellent dialyzing device, demonstrated the greatest increase in tobramycin clearance by increasing Q_d.

In contrast, an increase in URF from 0 to 20 ml/min resulted in a 240% increase in tobramycin clearance with all filter data combined. This was evident for every filter and even at large Q_d settings. Tobramycin clearance was greatest in the HF500, followed by the D30, HF250, D20 and finally the Biospal.

Tobramycin levels were determined at the filter inlet and outlet for each filter experiment. Plasma inlet tobramycin levels varied from 5 to

Table 1. Plasma tobramycin concentrations (mg/l)

	Biospal filter No. 1		Biospal filter No. 2		Biospal filter No. 3	
	inlet	outlet	inlet	outlet	inlet	outlet
Experiment 1	15.7	0.9	8.0	1.1	5.6	0.7
Experiment 2	15.4	1.1	8.3	1.0	5.6	0.7
Experiment 3	14.5	1.2	8.3	1.1	5.9	0.6

15 mg/l depending on when the reservoir was re-stocked with drug. For the HF500, HF250, D30 and D20 filters, the inlet-to-outlet tobramycin concentration difference was rarely greater than 2 mg/l, and usually the difference was <1 mg/l. The first three sets of samples for the three Biospal filters are displayed in table 1, demonstrating a major extraction of tobramycin from the plasma as it transisted the Biospal. Clearances were determined from dialysate measurements and tobramycin did not appreciably appear in the dialysate.

Tobramycin behaved predictably regarding its clearance in simulated CAVHD. Compared to urea and inulin, its clearance demonstrated small dependence on Q_d and larger dependence on UFR. Inulin clearance depended on UFR while urea clearance was affected by both Q_d and UFR [7].

Furthermore, major binding of tobramycin to AN69S membrane is suggested by the low dialysate measured clearance and the high extraction difference noted across the filter. This is consistent with the data of others [6, 8]. Our reservoir contained 15–45 mg of tobramycin and it is thought that the Biospal binds 10–20 mg.

References

1   Matzke GR, Halstenson CE, Keane WF: Hemodialysis elimination rates and clearance of gentamicin and tobramycin. Antimicrob Agents Chemother 1984;25:128–130.

2   Rumpf KW, Rieger J, Doht B, Ansorg R, Scheler F: Drug elimination by hemofiltration. J Dial 1977;1:677–688.

3   Basile C, Di Maggio A, Curino E, Scatizzi A: Pharmacokinetics of netilmicin in hypertonic hemodiafiltration and standard hemodialysis. Clin Nephrol 1985;24:305–309.

4   Golper TA, Wedel SK, Kaplan AA, Saad A-M, Donta ST: Drug removal during continuous arteriovenous hemofiltration: Theory and clinical observations. Int J Artif Organs 1985;8:307–312.

5   Golper TA, Saad A-MA: Gentamicin and phenytoin sieving through hollow-fiber polysulfone hemofilters. Kidney Int, 1986;30:937–943.

6   Kronfol NO, Lau AH, Barakat MM: Aminoglycoside binding to polyacrylonitrile hemofilter membranes during continuous hemofiltration. Trans ASAIO 1987;33:300–303.

7   Golper TA, Cigarran-Guldris S, Jenkins RD, Brier ME: The role of convection during simulated continuous arteriovenous hemodialysis; in Sieberth HG, Mann H, Stummvoll HK (eds): Continuous Hemofiltration. Contrib Nephrol. Basel, Karger, 1991, vol 93, pp 146–148.
8   Kraft D, Lode H: Elimination of ampicillin and gentamicin by hemofiltration. Klin Wochenschr 1979;57:195–196.

S. Cigarran-Guldris, MD, University of Louisville, 500 South Floyd Street, Louisville, KY 40292 (USA)

Sieberth HG, Mann H, Stummvoll HK (eds): Continuous Hemofiltration.
Contrib Nephrol. Basel, Karger, 1991, vol 93, pp 124–126

Pefloxacin and Metabolites Removal in Continuous Hemofiltration with Dialysis

D. Journois, D. Chanu, C. Drévillon, M. Dru, M. Ballereau, D. Safran

Réanimation chirurgicale, Hôpital Laënnec, Paris, France

Continuous venovenous hemodiafiltration (CVVHD) is being used increasingly for the treatment of acute renal failure. Drug handling during this technique is briefly mentioned. This study was undertaken to determine the clearance and the sieving characteristics of pefloxacin (P) and its two major metabolites (the bacteriologically active N-desmethyl-P and the inactive N-oxide-P) during CVVHD in vitro.

Material and Method

The experimental set-up is shown in figure 1. 450 ml of human citrate dextrose anticoagulated fresh blood, drawn from a patient with hemochromatosis, were used. Blood was circulated at 100 ml/min through a high-performance polyacrylonitrile hemofilter set (AN-69S, Hospal®) using a blood roller pump device (BSM22, Hospal®). Dialysate fluid (L2D, Hospal®) was circulated at three different flow rates (Q_{di}): 0, 500 and 1,000 ml/h. The dialysate and ultrafiltrate outflow was continuously regulated to obtain zero net ultrafiltration using a withdrawal pump. Temperature and ionic blood composition were controlled and kept within physiological values.

P and its two metabolites were added to reach usual therapeutic levels. For each of the experiments performed, two sets of simultaneous samples were obtained for HPLC determinations after 10 min of equilibration. Sieving (S) and clearance (Cl) coefficients have been calculated using the rigorous formula of Colton-Henderson [1] which uses arterial (C_a), venous (C_v) and ultrafiltrate concentrations (C_u) and flow rate (UFR): $S = 2 \times C_u/(C_a + C_v)$ and $Cl = C_u \times UFR/C_a$. Concentration values were corrected according to plasma protein levels: $C_i = $ Plasma drug concentration/$(1 - [$Total protein concentration $\times 0.0107])$ [2].

Results

The observed clearances and sieving coefficient are reported in table 1.

Discussion and Conclusion

Drugs bound to proteins will remain with the protein drug transit through the hemofilter. Only the unbound fraction of a drug has the potential for removal by ultrafiltration. P is approximately 20–30% protein

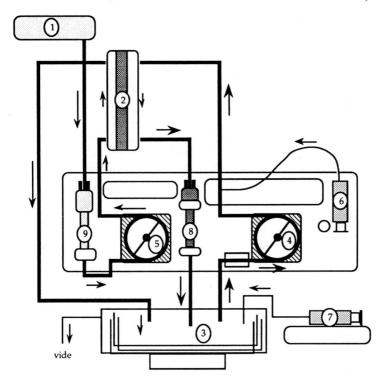

Fig. 1. Experimental set-up: 1 = dialysate reservoir; 2 = hemofiltration membrane; 3 = blood reservoir and ultrafiltrate collection bag; 4 = blood pump; 5 = dialysate pump; 6 = anticoagulation set; 7 = ultrafiltration compensation set; 8, 9 = air embolism protection set.

Table 1. Sieving and observed clearance of P, N-desmethyl-P and N-oxide-P at three different additional dialysis flow rates during continuous hemofiltration using a Hospal AN-69S flat hemofilter

	Dialysis rate ml/min	P ml/min	N-desmethyl-P ml/min	N-oxide-P ml/min
Clearances	0	6.8	7.1	9.9
	500	15.2	15.8	17.0
	1,000	15.0	14.7	18.5
Sieving coefficient		0.42	0.45	0.58

bound, this relatively low value, which is independent of the drug concentration [3], considered with P (and metabolites) low molecular weights should have provided high sieving coefficients. The two bacteriologically active forms (P and N-desmethyl-P) seem to have the same removal characteristics, whereas the inactive N-oxide-P metabolite may be better removed by CVVHD. This could be explained by a higher water solubility. These in vitro results show that at the blood flow used, clearances were proportionally related to the dialysate flow rate. A 500 ml/h dialysate flow rate added to convective transport approximately provides the P clearance observed in normal people. An accumulation of P and its metabolites is consequently avoided.

Although this study was clearly not designed to evaluate the possible displacement effects of uremia on P or metabolites bound to proteins, these data are helpful in estimating dose adjustments needed in patients with acute renal failure.

References

1   Colton CK, Henderson LW, Ford CA, Lysaght MJ: Kinetics of haemodiafiltration. I. In vitro transport characteristics of a hollow-fiber blood ultrafilter. J Lab Clin Med 1975;85:355–381.
2   Kronfol NO, Lau AH, Colon-Rivera J, Libertin C: Trans Am Soc Intern Organs 1986;32:85–87.
3   Montay G, Goueffon Y, Roquet F: Absorption, distribution, metabolic fate and elimination of pefloxacin mesylate in mice, rats, dogs, monkeys and humans. Antimicrob Agents Chemother 1984;25:463–472.

Dr. D. Journois, Réanimation chirurgicale, Hôpital Laënnec,
42, rue de Sèvres, F–75007 Paris (France)

Sieberth HG, Mann H, Stummvoll HK (eds): Continuous Hemofiltration.
Contrib Nephrol. Basel, Karger, 1991, vol 93, pp 127–130

Drug Dosage during Continuous Hemofiltration: Pharmacokinetics and Practical Implications

U.F. Kroh, M. Dehne, K. El Abed, K.D. Feußner, W. Hofmann, H. Lennartz

Department of Anesthesiology and Intensive Therapy, University of Marburg, FRG

Since the convective blood purification methods became routine in operative intensive therapy units (ITU), the pump-assisted continuous techniques have displaced CAVH for catabolic patients with multiorgan failure (MOF). With continuous volume controlled hemofiltration (CVHF) the elimination of soluta could be tuned to the metabolic requirement [1].

In order to perform optimized drug therapy, we installed a special drug-monitoring laboratory to receive pharmacokinetic data from CVHF and MOF patients. For cases where blood levels were not always available, a simple and practical dosage algorithm was developed for predictions. This should improve dosage for first estimations and changed organ functions.

Estimation of Drug Dosage

CVHF was performed as a postdilution technique with a polysulfone high flux filter (AV-600, Fresenius, Bad Homburg, FRG) and a blood pump (BMM10, Gambro Medizintechnik KG, München, FRG) to receive constant filtration rates ($Q_F = 20$–30 ml/min). The drug levels from serum and ultrafiltrate were determined by HPLC and FPIA. 143 paired pharmacokinetics (S/UF) were analyzed during steady-state conditions by a 2KM least-squares method (TOPFIT) [2]. Up to now, the kinetics of 15 drugs were investigated in 72 MOF/CVHF patients. Correct dosages were calculated as a standard for mean blood levels identical to normals [3]:

$$D = D_n \cdot \frac{V \cdot \tau \cdot k_{el}}{V_n \cdot \tau_n \cdot k_{eln}} \cdot \qquad (1)$$

The predictive algorithm was based on Dettli's assumptions for renal insufficiency [4]:

$$D = D_n \cdot \left(Q_o + \frac{1 - Q_o}{Cl_{crn}} \cdot Cl_{cr} \right), \qquad (2)$$

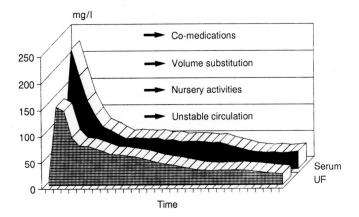

mg/l

- → Co-medications
- → Volume substitution
- → Nursery activities
- → Unstable circulation

Serum
UF

Time

Fig. 1. Concentration-time curves during CVHF piperacillin (4 g/30 min) (Q_F = 36 ml/ min). Influence factors on the precision of calculated drug sieving during hemofiltration. Simultaneous plot of serum and ultrafiltrate concentrations in a typical case from the ITU.

with $Cl_{cr} = Q_F$. The second term of equation 2 was suggested to be the CVHF-specific fraction of elimination. To correct for hemofiltration clearance, it had to be replaced with $Q_F \cdot S / V_n \cdot K_{eln}$. S (sieving coefficient) [5] was calculated from the AUC_F / AUC_P quotient, because this seemed to be more precise for ITU conditions: figure 1 shows some unavoidable influence factors on drug concentrations. These would falsify the results for S received from simple concentration quotients [6]. The first term of equation 2 was a drug-specific constant for the extrarenal elimination fraction Q_O (k_{nr}/k_{eln}). It was recalculated from kinetics as Q_x for each MOF/CVHF patient and drug. In completely unuric patients Q_x would reflect the remaining elimination capacity of the body. This induced us to compare Q_x and other kinetic data (volume of distribution V) with clinical parameters like scores and laboratory data to enable for predictions. The new drug-dosage formula for MOF/CVHF patients resulted as:

$$D = D_n \cdot \left(Q_x + \frac{Q_F \cdot S}{V_n \cdot k_{eln}} \right),$$ (3)

this should facilitate clinicians to predict individualized dosage concerning the extracorporal device as well as the present state of illness.

Results

As presumed, the dosage of 11 investigated drugs should be reduced during CVHF (table 1). But this was not only dependent on Q_F or the sieving coefficient: S was in good accordance with the normal free fraction:

Table 1. Drug dosage during hemofiltration ($Q_F = 20-30$ ml/min); medians of (n) paired pharmacokinetic analyses (mg/24 h/70 kg BW)

Drug	n	Normal		Equation 1		Equation 3	Clinical dose
Amikacin	4	1,050	*	280		273	$1-2 \times 250$
Netilmicin	11	420	**	139		136	$1 \times 100-150$
Tobramycin	10	350	**	115		107	1×100
Vancomycin	10	2,000	**	645		653	$1-2 \times 500$
Ceftazidim	11	6,000	**	1,675		1,622	$2 \times 1,000$
Cefotaxim	13	12,000	**	3,235		3,380	$2 \times 2,000$
Ciprofloxacin	9	400	**	98	*	167	1×200
Imipenem	10	4,000	**	1,754		1,614	$3-4 \times 500$
Metronidazol	7	2,100	**	1,376		1,860	$3-4 \times 500$
Piperacillin	17	24,000	**	10,271		9,737	$3 \times 4,000$
Digitoxin	9	0.065		0.05		0.06	1×0.05
Digoxin	9	0.29	**	0.07		0.10	1×0.10
Phenobarbital	8	233		330	**	480	$2-4 \times 100$
Phenytoin	2	524		453		364	$1-2 \times 250$
Theophyllin	12	720		889	*	745	$600-900$

*p < 0.05; **p < 0.01, Wilcoxon's rank test.

$r = 0.926$, $p < 0.0001$, $n = 15$ (means), and $r = 0.663$, $p < 0.0001$, $n = 143$ (individuals).

Q_x ranged between 0 and 3.4 for all drugs metabolized normally. It correlated with one score of illness for CTX ($r = 0.695$, $p = 0.008$, $n = 13$), CIP ($r = 0.639$, $p = 0.064$, $n = 9$), PIP ($r = 0.385$, $p = 0.126$, $n = 17$), PHB ($r = 0.825$, $p = 0.019$, $n = 8$), and THE ($r = 0.705$, $p = 0.011$, $n = 12$). For PHB and THE enzyme induction could be assumed ($Q_x > 1$). The plot of the APACHE II score on Q_x cleared for Q_o (fig. 2) demonstrates high significant but not very specific correlation of the clinic with the drug elimination.

The relative volumes of distribution (V/V_n) ranged within 0.2 and 2.5. Obviously here there was no general connection with any documented clinical parameter.

The final correlation of the dosage predictions (eq. 3) on pharmacokinetics (eq. 1) was $r = 0.950$, $p < 0.00001$, $n = 126$ with a prediction precision of 79% (34–98%) for the medians.

Discussion and Conclusion

Convective blood purification allowed simple and precise predictions for the artificial part of drug elimination. The extra-renal fraction depended on factors that could be taken bedsides without blood level measurements. Nevertheless, wide-ranging scales of pharmacokinetic parameters were

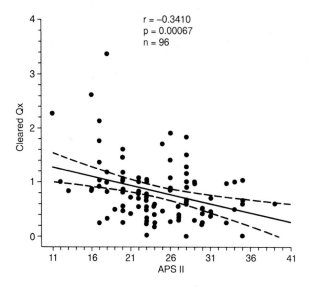

Fig. 2. Regression of the APACHE II score [7] on the nonrenal elimination fraction of drugs Q_x with $Q_o > 0.2$ [4] cleared for Q_o (Q_x/Q_o).

observed (k_{nr}, V). This would enforce us to examine blood levels from all critically ill patients receiving toxic drugs. For the others, a dose up to 50% higher than predicted should be sufficient as long as bayesian forecastings are not available. Now we are looking forward to integrate the results into a program concerning the specific parameters of the critically ill.

References
1   Kroh U, Hofmann W, Dehne M, El Abed K, Lennartz H: Dosisanpassung von Pharmaka während kontinuierlicher Hämofiltration. Anaesthesist 1989;38:225–232.
2   Bozler G, Heinzel G, Koss FW, Wolf M: Modellentwicklung in der Pharmakokinetik, I. Allgemeine Strategie. Drug Res 1977;27:897–900.
3   Keller F, Mohlzahn M, Vöhringer HF: Pharmakotherapie bei Niereninsuffizienz. Inn Med 1982;9:377–381.
4   Dettli L, Galeazzi RL: Pharmakokinetische Grundlagen der Arzneimittelforschung. Arzneimittelkomp Schweiz 1986;2:2051–2074.
5   Golper TA, Wedel SK, Kaplan AA, Saad AM, Donta ST, Paganini EP: Drug removal during continuous arteriovenous hemofiltration: Theory and clinical observation. Int J Artif Organs 1985;8:307–312.
6   Lee CC, Marbury TC: Drug therapy in patients undergoing hemodialysis: Clinical pharmocokinetic considerations. Clin Pharmacokinet 1984;9:42–66.
7   Knaus WA, Draper EA, Wagner JE: Apache II: A severity of disease classification system. Crit Care Med 1985;13:818–829.

Dr. U.F. Kroh, Abteilung für Anästhesie und Intensivtherapie am Klinikum der Philipps-Universität Marburg, Baldinger Strasse 1, D–W–3550 Marburg (FRG)

Sieberth HG, Mann H, Stummvoll HK (eds): Continuous Hemofiltration.
Contrib Nephrol. Basel, Karger, 1991, vol 93, pp 131–134

Pharmacokinetics of Imipenem/Cilastatin during Continuous Arteriovenous Hemofiltration

M. Przechera, D. Bengel, T. Risler

Department of Nephrology, University of Tübingen, FRG

Patients with acute renal failure undergoing continuous arteriovenous hemofiltration (CAVH) often require antibiotic therapy because of additional (nosocomial) infections. Therapy of these infections is most efficient with newly developed high potential β-lactam antibiotics with a widened spectrum in the gram-negative range. We therefore investigated the pharmacokinetics of imipenem and the dehydropeptidase inhibitor cilastatin during CAVH treatment.

Material and Methods

Six intensive-care patients (1 woman, 5 men), aged 22–65 years (mean 53.5 years) with acute renal failure were included in the study. They underwent CAVH because of a renal clearance less than 10 ml/min. There was no intermittent hemodialysis. All patients suffered from additional, often nosocomial infections and needed antibiotic therapy. None of them had known allergy to β-lactam antibiotics.

Study Design

After the beginning of hemofiltration all patients received a daily dose of 2 times 500/500 mg imipenem/cilastatin. The relative dosage ranged between 6.4 and 8.9 mg/kg body weight. The spontaneous filtration flow ranged between 4.9 and 9.8 ml/min (mean 6.6 ml/min).

The high pressure liquid chromatography (HPLC) technique by Myers and Blumer [1] was used to determine plasma and ultrafiltrate levels of imipenem and cilastatin.

Blood samples were drawn from the arterial line of the CAVH. Two hours after the end of infusion samples of the venous line were used to determine the sieving coefficients.

CAVH was performed using a capillary hemofilter.

Hemofilter: Polyamide capillary hemofilter FH 66 GAMBRO: surface area, 0.6 m²; wall thickness, 50 μm; inner diameter, 215 μm. Imipenem: MW 317.37 daltons; PPB, 10–25%. Cilastatin: MW 380.43 daltons; PPB, 35–45%.

Results

Pharmacokinetic Analysis. The initial plasma concentration Coβ (extrapolated initial concentrations of the real volume of distribution) and the elimination constant Ceβ were calculated using linear regression after transforming the data into logarithmic values.

Using the two-compartment model the following values for imipenem (cilastatin) were obtained:

$$\text{Terminal excretion half-life:} \quad t\tfrac{1}{2}\beta = \frac{\ln 2}{Ce\beta} = 2\,\text{h}\ 49\,\text{min.}$$
$$(14\,\text{h}\ 39\,\text{min})$$

The volume of distribution of the central compartment was calculated using the following equation (W = weight):

$$V_{abs} = \frac{D}{Co\beta} \qquad V_{rel} = \frac{V_{abs}}{W}.$$

Imipenem: $V_{abs} = 34.8\,1 \pm 8.90$; $V_{rel} = 0.47\,1/\text{kg}/W \pm 0.16$.
Cilastatin: $V_{abs} = 17.5\,1 \pm 4.82$; $V_{rel} = 0.25\,1/\text{kg}/W \pm 0.08$.

The mean clearances-CAVH were 6.49 ml/min for imipenem and 4.7 ml/min for cilastatin with an average filtration rate of 6.6 ml/min.

To determine the sieving coefficients (SC), the following equation was used:

$$SC = \frac{CuF}{\dfrac{C_{in} + C_{out}}{2}}.$$

Imipenem: $SC = 1.13 \pm 0.12$. Cilastatin: $SC = 0.77 \pm 0.08$.

Because theoretically all substances with a $MW \leqslant 10{,}000$ daltons can freely pass the hemofiltration membrane the expected SC of a pharmacon should equal the nonprotein-bound fraction.

Side Effects. The antibiotic therapy with imipenem/cilastatin was well tolerated by all patients with no side reactions.

Discussion

In patients with normal renal function the clearance of imipenem (renal excretion and metabolism, nonrenal metabolism) equals the value of clearance of cilastatin [3].

In patients with renal insufficiency the elimination half-life of imipenem is prolonged because only the nonrenal metabolism in plasma continues [4, 5]. The total clearance of cilastatin is reduced markedly

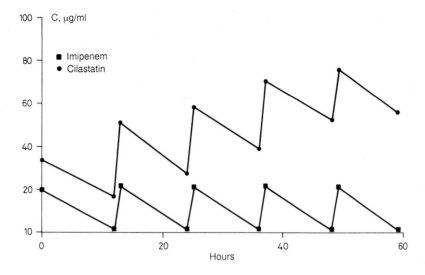

Fig. 1. Plasma levels of the exponentially eliminated pharmacons imipenem/cilastatin during continued intermittent application of equal doses (500 mg/500 mg). Application intervals = 12 h.

because normally the renal route (excretion and acetylation) is the major elimination way.

During hemodialysis only about 60% ($t_\frac{1}{2}$ = 3.7 h) of the initial dose of cilastatin is eliminated compared to 80–90% ($t_\frac{1}{2}$ = 1.5 h) elimination of imipenem [2]. Supplemental doses are required after dialysis, which will lead to the accumulation of cilastatin. The clearance by CAVH of both substances is low (imipenem 6.49; cilastatin 4.7) and correlates with low ultrafiltrate flow rate (6.6 ml/h).

With a dosage schedule of 500 mg/500 mg imipenem/cilastatin twice a day given i.v., there was no accumulation of imipenem (fig. 1). The therapeutic plasma level of 4 mg/l (minimal inhibitory plasma concentration), however, is maintained over 6 h only. Therefore, the application interval concerning imipenem should be shortened.

In contrast, the elimination half-line of cilastatin is 14.39 h. This leads to a maximum cumulation level of 114.6 mg/l after 4.5 half-lives. The mean equilibrium concentration level was 85 mg/l. These levels remain constant during the above dosing schedule. Till now, there is no clinical evidence of other than nephroprotective effects of the dehydropeptidase inhibitor cilastatin even at such high doses.

Conclusions

After application of imipenem blood levels exceeded the minimal inhibitory concentration of 4.0 mg/l for 6 h only. Therefore, the application intervals need to be shortened. In contrast to patients with normal renal function, we found a considerable dissociation of kinetics of both pharmacons and a cumulation of cilastatin.

References

1   Myers CM, Blumer JF: Determination of imipenem and cilastatin in serum by high-pressure liquid chromatography. Antimicrob Agents Chemother 1984;26:78–81.
2   Berman SJ, Sugihara JG, Nakamura JM: Multiple study of imipenem/cilastatin in patients with end stage renal disease undergoing long term hemodialysis. Am J Med 1985;78:105–108.
3   Drusano GL, Standiford HC: Pharmacokinetic profile of imipenem/cilastatin in normal volunteers. Am J Med 1985;78(suppl 6a):47–53.
4   Verbist L, Veerpooten GA, Giuliano RA, Debroe ME, Buntinx AP, Entwistle LA, Jones KH: Pharmacokinetics and tolerance after repeated doses of imipenem/cilastatin in patients with severe renal failure. J Antimicrob. Chemother 1986;18(suppl E):115–120.
5   Gibson TP, Demetriades JL, Bland JA: Imipenem/Cilastatin: Pharmacokinetic profile in renal insufficiency. Am J Med 1985;78(suppl 6a):54–61.

Dr. M. Przechera, Medical Clinic III, University of Tübingen, Otfried-Müller-Strasse 10, D–W–7400 Tübingen (FRG)

Sieberth HG, Mann H, Stummvoll HK (eds): Continuous Hemofiltration.
Contrib Nephrol. Basel, Karger, 1991, vol 93, pp 135–139

Elimination of Vancomycin in Patients on Continuous Arteriovenous Hemodialysis

Petra Reetze-Bonorden, Joachim Böhler, Christoph Kohler,
Peter Schollmeyer, Erich Keller

Department of Nephrology, University of Freiburg, FRG

Continuous arteriovenous hemodialysis (CAVHD) [1], a modification of continuous arteriovenous hemofiltration [2], has been accepted as an alternative for the treatment of acute renal failure (ARF) in intensive care patients. However, only little is known about drug elimination during CAVHD [3, 4]. Basic pharmacokinetic drug data and the characteristics of continuous extracorporeal dialysis led to the assumption that vancomycin removal during CAVHD could be clinically relevant [5]. Because pharmacokinetics of vancomycin during CAVHD had not been published previously, this study was designed to obtain pharmacokinetic data and develop dosage guidelines.

Materials and Methods

Patients and Methods. Seven intensive care patients (mean age 61.7 ± 2.0 years, 3 females, 4 males) with ARF were investigated. Four patients were anuric (<100 ml urine/day), 3 had residual diuresis between 200 and 750 ml/day. One gram of vancomycin, dissolved in 250 ml normal saline, was infused into a central venous catheter over a period of 1 h for treatment of infection.

A polyacrylonitrile parallel-plate hemodialyzer was used (AN69S, Hospal[R], 0.43 m^2 surface area) for CAVHD. The dialysate flow rate was held constant at 1 liter/h by use of an infusion pump. To study vancomycin pharmacokinetics during CAVHD, repeated blood samples were drawn from the arterial line of the extracorporeal circuit, from dialysate and filtrate mixture (DF), and if present from urine. Blood was centrifuged immediately after drawing. All samples were stored at $-70\,°C$ until analysis. The study continued until the patients reached subtherapeutic drug plasma levels ($<5\,\mu g/ml$) [6]. Vancomycin plasma levels were determined by fluorescence polarization immunoassay (TDx Vancomycin[R]; Abbott, USA) [7].

Pharmacokinetics. The plasma concentration time course of vancomycin was analyzed according to a two-compartment open model (method of residuals [8]). The elimination constant (β) was calculated by log linear regression analysis of the terminal log linear portion of the plasma level time curve. Division of $\ln 2$ by β gave the elimination half-life of vancomycin ($t_{1/2}$). The area under the plasma level-time curve (AUC_{0-t}) was estimated using

Table 1. Pharmacokinetic data of vancomycin in patients (n = 7) on CAVHD

Volume of distribution (V_d), l	77.8 ± 8.8
Elimination half-life ($t_{1/2}$), h	56.3 ± 9.0
Clearance, ml/min	
Total body (Cl_B)	17.1 ± 1.9
CAVHD clearance (Cl_{CAVHD})	8.1 ± 1.2
Renal clearance (n = 3) (Cl_R)	2.7 ± 0.5

the linear trapezoidal rule and extrapolated to infinity by dividing the last pharmacon drug concentration value by β ($AUC_{0-\infty}$). Division of the administered dose by $AUC_{0-\infty}$ gave the total body clearance (Cl_B). The volume of distribution was estimated by dividing Cl_B by β. The removal of drug by CAVHD was determined by multiplying the concentrration of the drug in DF by DF-volume. The CAVHD-vancomycin clearance (Cl_{CAVHD}) was calculated by dividing the amount of vancomycin removed in DF by the corresponding AUC_{0-t}[8]. Data are given as mean $\pm$ SEM.

Results

The mean time of observation after vancomycin application was 92.8 ± 17.0 h. Because of interruptions, e.g. for replacement of the filter after clotting, the time on CAVHD during the observation period was 86.9 ± 14.4 h. The dialysate flow measured 16.7 ml/min and the filtrate flow 2.7 ± 0.3 ml/min. Thus the mean DF rate was 19.4 ml/min, corresponding to a creatinine and urea clearance of 19.3 ± 0.8 or 19.3 ± 1.0 ml/min, respectively. During treatment with CAVHD, serum creatinine measured 2.8 ± 0.3 mg/dl, while serum urea was 107.0 ± 11.0 mg/dl.

Pharmacokinetic parameters of vancomycin are given in table 1. The Cl_B was 17.1 ± 1.9 ml/min resulting in a weekly clearance of 172,368 ml. Cl_{CAVHD} measured 8.1 ± 1.2 ml/min or 81,648 ml/week. Thus the extracorporeal clearance of vancomycin reached nearly 50% of the Cl_B.

Figure 1 shows a typical vancomycin plasma level and DF level time curve in 1 patient. Due to distribution, vancomycin plasma levels rapidly declined during the first 4 h, according to a two-compartment open model. Thereafter, thus during the elimination phase, a less rapid decline continued, because of a high Cl_{CAVHD} of vancomycin. Plasma concentrations reached subtherapeutic drug levels after 2.8 ± 0.3 days (range 1.7–3.9).

Discussion

Vancomycin has long been regarded as nondialyzable and it was common practice to applicate 1 g of vancomycin per week in patients requiring dialysis [9, 10]. For highly permeable membranes, however,

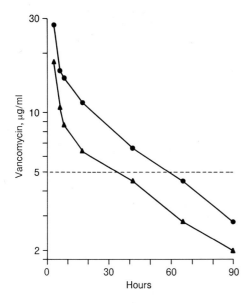

Fig. 1. Drug concentration in plasma (●) and dialysate/filtrate (▲) after intravenous infusion of 1 g of vancomycin during CAVHD in 1 patient (No. 6). Dotted line indicates subtherapeutic range for plasma levels.

high clearance of the drug has been demonstrated [11–14]. Continuous arteriovenous dialysis provides a lower creatinine clearance per minute but clinically relevant drug elimination may occur due to the continuous nature of the procedure [5].

In this study creatinine and urea clearance (19.3 ml/min) were almost identical to the dialysate/filtrate flow rate (19.4 ml/min), due to a more than 99% saturation of the dialysis solution with these substances. Vancomycin clearance (8.1 ml/min) averaged only 42% of creatinine and urea clearance (fig. 2), probably because of the larger molecular weight of the drug (MW 1,448 [10]). Although the removal of the drug per minute is limited, weekly vancomycin clearance is higher in CAVHD than in intermittent hemodialysis (HD). The weekly clearance by CAVHD was about twice the rate seen in chronic HD with high flux dialysis membranes (HD: 35,844 ml/week; CAVHD: 81,648 ml/week [14]). The Cl_{CAVHD} accounted for nearly 50% of total body clearance. As a consequence, the elimination half-life of vancomycin was markedly lower in patients on CAVHD than in patients on chronic HD ($t_{1/2}$ 90.3 h [14]).

The volume of distribution was elevated by about 75% in these intensive care patients compared to chronic uremic subjects [14]. This likely

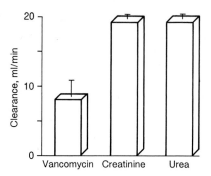

Fig. 2. Mean clearance rates (n = 7) of vancomycin, creatinine, and urea by CAVHD.

explains the low plasma concentrations found at the end of the initial distribution phase. An increase in the volume of distribution has been demonstrated for many drugs in critically ill patients, possibly due to an enhanced extracellular volume and alterations in protein binding [15, 16].

The enhanced volume of distribution and the high clearance rate of vancomycin by continuous dialysis both contribute to a rapid decline of plasma concentrations to levels below the therapeutic range of 5 μg/ml. Thus, the usual dosing recommendation of 1 g of vancomycin per week as in chronic HD patients [10, 14] will not suffice for patients with ARF treated with CAVHD. These pharmacokinetic data suggest that daily determinations of the drug levels are needed to adjust dosing.

References

1   Geronemus R, Schneider N: Continuous arteriovenous haemodialysis: a new modality for treatment of acute renal failure. Trans Am Soc Artif Intern Organs 1984;30:610–613.
2   Kramer P, Wigger W, Rieger J, Mattheai D, Scheler F: Arteriovenous haemofiltration: a new and simple method for treatment of overhydrated patients resistant to diuretics. Klin Wochenschr 1977;55:1121–1122.
3   Davies SP, Fahey M, Brown EA, Kox W: Pharmacokinetics of ceftazidime in patients with acute renal failure (ARF) treated by continuous arteriovenous haemodialysis (CAVHD). Abstr 16th Congr Chemother, Jerusalem, June 1989.
4   Kronfol NO, Adams LJ, Powell SS, Lau AH: Drug removal in continuous arteriovenous hemodialysis (CAVHD). Abstr 18th Annu Scient Meet National Kidney Foundation, 1988.
5   Reetze-Bonorden P, Böhler J, Kohler C, Schollmeyer P, Keller E: Arzneimitteltherapie bei kontinuierlichen Entgiftungsverfahren; in Keller E (ed): Kontinuierliche Filtrations- und Dialyseverfahren in der Intensivmedizin. Lengerich, Pabst Verlag, 1990.
6   Geraci JE, Hermans PE: Vancomycin. Mayo Clin Proc 1983;58:88–91.
7   Schwenzer KS, Chao-Huei JW, Anhalt JP: Automated fluorescence polarisation immunoassay for monitoring vancomycin. Ther Drug Monit 1983;5:341–345.

8   Rowland M, Tozer TN (eds): Clinical Pharmacokinetics. Concepts and Applications, ed 2. Philadelphia, Lea & Febiger, 1989.
9   Appel GB, Given DB, Levine LR, Cooper GL: Vancomycin and the kidney. Am J Kidney Dis 1986;8:75–80.
10   Matzke GR, Zhanel GG, Guay DRP: Clinical pharmacokinetics of vancomycin. Clin Pharmacokinet 1986;11:257–282.
11   Keller F: Vancomycin administration to hemodialysis patients. Clin Nephrol 1988;30:173.
12   de Bock V, Verbeelen D, Maes V, Sennesael J: Pharmacokinetics of vancomycin in patients undergoing hemodialysis and hemofiltration. Nephrol Dial Transplant 1989;4:635–639.
13   Lanese DM, Alfrey PS, Molitoris BA: Markedly increased clearance of vancomycin during hemodialysis using polysulfone dialyzers. Kidney Int 1989;35:1409–1412.
14   Böhler J, Reetze-Bonorden P, Keller E, Kramer A, Schollmeyer PJ: Elimination of vancomycin with highly permeable dialysis membranes. Abstr 27th ISN Congr, Tokyo 1990.
15   Craig WA, Suh B: Changes in protein binding during disease. Scand J Infect Dis 1978; suppl 14:239–244.
16   Bodenham A, Shelly MP, Park GR: The altered pharmacokinetics and pharmacodynamics of drugs commonly used in critically ill patients. Clin Pharmacokinet 1988;14:347–373.

Dr. Petra Reetze-Bonorden, Medizinische Universitätsklinik, Abteilung Innere Medizin, Dialysestation, Kilianstrasse 5, D–W–7800 Freiburg i. Br. (FRG)

Sieberth HG, Mann H, Stummvoll HK (eds): Continuous Hemofiltration.
Contrib Nephrol. Basel, Karger, 1991, vol 93, pp 140–142

Comparitive Vancomycin Kinetics in Intensive Care Unit Patients with Acute Renal Failure: Intermittent Hemodialysis versus Continuous Hemofiltration Hemodialysis

Peter H. Slugg, Marcus T. Haug, Cindy Bosworth, Emil P. Paganini

Cleveland Clinic Foundation, Cleveland, Ohio, USA

Dosing vancomycin to achieve optimal drug levels can be difficult in the presence of acute (ARF) or chronic (CRF) renal failure as the kidneys are the primary source of drug elimination [1]. Continuous hemofiltration (CAVH), a hemofiltration technique frequently used to support intensive care unit (ICU) patients, has shown to alter vancomycin elimination [2]. Further, dosing medications in the ICU setting is frequently complicated by an unpredictable variability of pharmacokinetic estimates including elimination [3]. Shortly after we instituted assisted pharmacokinetic dosing by the Clinical Pharmacology Service (CPS) it became apparent that ICU patients receiving support with CAVH or continuous hemodialysis (CAVHD) had substantial alterations in vancomycin disposition in comparison to those receiving intermittent hemodialysis (IHD). This report summarizes our experience and preliminary findings.

Methods

ICU patients with ARF receiving IHD or CAVH/CAVHD support seen by the CPS for vancomycin dosing were evaluated. Clinical and laboratory data were obtained on a daily basis and recorded in the CPS data base. Pharmacokinetic parameters were calculated utilizing measured serum drug levels and a bayesian dosing system with a two-compartment open model (USC-PAK). Statistical calculations were made using Student's paired testing and regression analysis for trends.

Results

Eighteen patients with ARF were included (11 males, 7 females; mean height 173.6 cm; mean body weight 78.0 kg; mean body surface area 2.0 m^2). IHD (8 patients) consisted of 3.76 ± 0.5 h at Q_b 275 ml/min removing 2.15 ± 1.31 liters/run over $3.7 \pm$ sessions/week using a cuprophane membrane (Allegro; Baxter Corp., Round Lakes, Ill./USA).

Table 1. Vancomycin dosing and serum levels

	Hemodialysis	CAVH/CAVHD	p value
Mean dose, mg	961.3 ± 255.5	1,121.4 ± 204.2	<0.05
Mean dose interval, h	123.1 ± 72.7	63.1 ± 28.3	<0.05
Peak level, μg/ml	32.4 ± 6.7	28.8 ± 3.6	NS
	(21.6 − 44.8)	(22.8 − 36.1)	
Trough level, μg/ml	14.2 ± 6.0	11.1 ± 2.8	<0.08

Table 2. Vancomycin pharmacokinetics

	Hemodialysis	CAVH/CAVHD	p value
$t_{1/2\alpha}$, h	0.8 ± 0.6	0.8 ± 0.5	NS
$t_{1/2\beta}$, h	158.9 ± 131.7	70.7 ± 24.5	<0.005
Volume of distribution[a], 1/kg	0.30 ± 0.13	0.25 ± 0.12	NS
	(0.11 − 0.63)	(0.12 − 0.53)	
KCP/h	0.7327 ± 0.1280	0.8174 ± 0.3940	NS
	(0.0900 − 1.6340)	(0.0592 − 1.748)	
KPC/h	0.2809 ± 0.1279	0.3109 ± 0.0953	NS
	(0.0400 − 0.5362)	(0.1143 − 0.5354)	
Kel/h	0.0232 ± 0.0166	0.458 ± 0.0239	<0.01
	(0.0090 − 0.1170)	(0.0171 − 0.1312)	
Cp average, μg/ml	20.5 ± 7.9	17.3 ± 3.0	<0.05
	(14.5 − 45.0)	(12.4 − 25.2)	

[a]Central compartment only. $t_{1/2\alpha}$ = Alpha half life; $t_{1/2\beta}$ = beta half life; KCP = constant for central to peripheral compartment; KPC = constant for peripheral to central compartment; Kel = elimination constant; Cp average = average concentration.

CAVH (9 patients) produced 11.99 ml/min exchange with an asymmetric polyamide membrane (FH-55/65, Gambro Corp.) and either bicarbonate- or acetate-base replacement made in our pharmacy; average filter life was 90.25 h. CAVHD (3 patients) utilized Dianeal 1.5% dialysate (Baxter Corp.) at 13.49 ml/min, and achieving an average 123 ml/h ultrafiltrate using a polyacrylonitrile membrane (Asahi Corp., Tokyo, Japan) with an average filter life of 52 h. There were 32 dosings on IHD and 14 for CAVH/CAVHD. Results of dosing and drug levels are shown in table 1 and pharmacokinetic parameters are summarized in table 2. Patients on

CAVH/CAVHD received larger doses at shorter intervals. There was no difference in volume of distribution; the beta half-life was markedly shorter in comparison to IHD patients.

Discussion

Although IHD with conventional membranes does not remove vancomycin to any appreciable degree, our experience, as well as others [4, 5], has shown that treatment with CAVH/CAVHD can substantially alter vancomycin disposition and thereby offers the potential for inappropriate drug dosing and suboptimal drug therapy. Our concurrent CPS monitoring/dosing system has also clearly demonstrated that critically ill patients also display substantial but predictable alterations in vancomycin disposition.

Based on our results it is our recommendation that patients with renal failure on vancomycin with optimal levels the dosing interval should be reduced in half when CAVH/CAVHD is started. For patients on CAVH/CAVHD who have optimal vancomycin levels, the vancomycin dosing interval should be doubled when CAVH/CAVHD is discontinued. Pharmacokinetic calculations with dosing support may be helpful for optimizing drug therapy.

References

1   Matzke GR, Zhanel GG, Guay DRP: Clinical pharmacokinetics of vancomycin. Clin Pharmacokinet 1986;11:257–282.
2   Matzke GR, O'Connell, MB, Collins AJ, Keshaviah PR: Disposition of vancomycin during hemofiltration. Clin Pharmacol Ther 1986;40:425–430.
3   Haug MT, Slugg P, Lockrem J, Byrnes J: High dose aminoglycoside therapy in surgical ICU patients (abstract) Clin Pharmacol Ther 1990;47:208.
4   Bellomo R, Ernest D, Parkin G, Boyce N: Clearance of vancomycin during continuous arteriovenous hemodiafiltration. Crit Care Med 1990;18:181–183.
5   Lau AH, Kronfol NO, John E: Increased vancomycin elimination with continuous hemofiltration. Trans Am Soc Artif Intern Organs 1987;33:772–774.

Peter H. Slugg, MD, Head, Section of Clinical Pharmacology, Cleveland Clinic Foundation, 9500 Euclid Avenue, Cleveland, OH 44195 (USA)

Sieberth HG, Mann H, Stummvoll HK (eds): Continuous Hemofiltration.
Contrib Nephrol. Basel, Karger, 1991, vol 93, pp 143–145

Continuous Arteriovenous Hemodiafiltration: Predicting the Clearance of Drugs

M.C. Vos, H.H. Vincent

Department of Internal Medicine I, University Hospital, Rotterdam, The Netherlands

In continuous arteriovenous hemodiafiltration (CAVHD) very high solute clearance rates can safely be obtained. These high clearance rates may have consequences for the plasma concentration of drugs. For some drugs, the influence of CAVHD will be irrelevant. In case of a very high molecular weight or a high protein binding, CAVHD clearance is generally negligible. With digoxin, due to the big volume of distribution, the change in plasma drug concentration, that results from CAVHD, occurs slowly. Dose adjustments may be deferred until results of repeated determination of plasma drug concentration have been received. For drugs that are rapidly cleared from the blood by nonrenal mechanisms, the contribution of CAVHD is likely to be small. On the other hand, there are a number of antibiotics that are normally excreted almost exclusively by the kidney. These include the aminoglycosides, cephalosporins, ciprofloxacin and the imipenem/cilastatin combination. With these drugs, the contribution of CAVHD to the clearance may be important enough to warrant prompt dose adjustments. Information on the rate of excretion by the hemofilter is needed in order to determine what dose adjustments have to be made.

Methods

Our new mathematical model of hemodiafiltration [1] was used to analyze the clearance of drugs by CAVHD. Patients were treated for renal failure and sepsis and/or circulatory, respiratory or neurological instability. Antibiotics were given as clinically indicated. We used the 0.6 m^2 AN-69 capillary hemofilter (Multiflow-60®; Hospal France). Filters had been used for 0–6 days. Average blood flow rate was 130 ml/min. Concentrations were determined in the arterial line and in the spent ultrafiltrate/dialysate after equilibration at dialysate flow rates of 0 liter/h (CAVH) and of 1 and 3 liters/h (CAVHD). The analysis included calculation of sieving coefficients (concentration in filtrate compared to that in plasma), clearance, and diffusive mass transfer coefficients (K_d) of creatinine and drugs. The filter condition was characterized by the blood pressure drop over the filter and the membrane index of

Table 1. Sieving coefficients and CAVHD clearance rates

Drug	n	Sieving coefficient	CAVHD clearance, ml/min	
			Q_d 1 liter/h	Q_d 3 liters/h
Tobramycin	11	0.90 (0.87–0.99)	24 (22–29)	32 (31–37)
Vancomycin	2	0.70 (0.67–0.73)	21 (19–29)	24 (17–30)
Cefuroxime	10	0.86 (0.67–0.97)	19 (8–48)	35 (11–49)
Cefotaxime	6	0.79 (0.64–0.94)	17 (12–23)	26 (20–33)
Imipenem	8	1.07 (0.88–1.60)	21 (11–31)	33 (16–49)
Ceftazidime	9	0.94 (0.82–1.00)	17 (14–18)	24 (19–27)

Table 2. Estimated plasma half-lives

Drug	Estimated plasma half-life, h				
	normal	anuric	CAVH	CAVHD 1 l/h	CAVHD 3 l/h
Tobramycin	3	56	15	7	5
Vancomycin	8	120	30	13	10
Cefuroxime	2	17	8	5	3
Cefotaxime	1	3	2	2	1
Imipenem	1	4	3	3	2
Ceftazidime	2	20	11	8	6

ultrafiltration [1]. The observed relationship between solute molecular weight and K_d was used together with data on the filter condition to predict drug clearance in individual cases. Using literature data on endogenous clearance rates and on distribution volumes, we estimated plasma drug concentration half-lives.

Results

Data are presented as median (range). Sieving coefficients and CAVHD clearance rates are given in table 1. Observed and predicted values of drug clearance are shown in figure 1. Estimated half-lives are given in table 2.

Discussion

For drugs with a molecular weight < 800 daltons, the sieving coefficient corresponded with protein binding. CAVH clearance may be

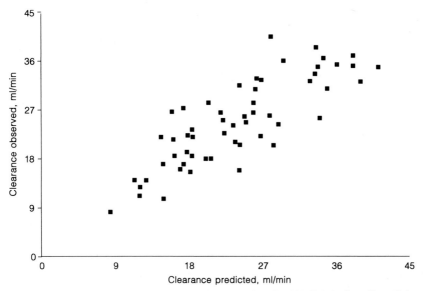

Fig. 1. Drug clearance prediction in CAVHD, using the AN-69 0.6 m² capillary dialyzer at dialysate flow rates of 1 and of 3 liters/h. Data were obtained for cefotaxime, ceftazidime, cefuroxime, ciprofloxacin, imipenem, tobramycin, vancomycin.

calculated from ultrafiltration rate and sieving coefficient. CAVHD clearance was rather variable (table 1). However, by taking filter condition and ultrafiltration rate into account, a fairly accurate prediction of drug clearance was feasible (fig. 1). The influence of CAVH and CAVHD on plasma half-life was most pronounced for tobramycin and vancomycin (table 2). For this class of drugs, dose adjustments are certainly needed. Also for the cephalosporins, failure to take the clearance by CAVHD into account may lead to inadequate plasma drug levels and therapeutic failure.

Reference

1   Vincent HH, van Ittersum FJ, Akcahuseyin E, Vos MC, van Duyl WA, Schalekamp MADH: Solute transport in continuous arterio-venous hemodiafiltration. A new mathematical model applied to clinical data. Blood Purif, 1990;8:149–159.

Dr. H.H. Vincent, University Hospital Dijkzigt, Room Bd 338, Dr Molewaterplein 40, NL–3015 GD Rotterdam (The Netherlands)

Technical Aspects of Solute Transport

Sieberth HG, Mann H, Stummvoll HK (eds): Continuous Hemofiltration..
Contrib Nephrol. Basel, Karger, 1991, vol 93, pp 146–148

The Role of Convection during Simulated Continuous Arteriovenous Hemodialysis

Thomas A. Golper, Secundino Cigarran-Guldris, Randall D. Jenkins, Michael E. Brier

University of Louisville, Ky., USA

Continuous arteriovenous hemodialysis (CAVHD) developed as an offspring from continuous arteriovenous hemofiltration [1]. CAVHD removes solute by diffusion; ultrafiltration is utilized for volume control. Diffusion removes small solutes while convection favors the removal of larger solutes. We investigated solute transport in simulated CAVHD while diffusion and convection were both maximized by increasing dialysate flow rate (Q_d) and ultrafiltration rate (UFR), respectively.

Materials and Methods

Materials and methods are described in more detail in our companion paper [2]. CAVHD was simulated with calibrated pumps for plasma, dialysate inflow and dialysate outflow. Plasma contained urea, tobramycin and inulin, and was pumped at 60 ml/min for all experiments. Q_d was either 15, 30 or 60 ml/min and UFR was either 0, 5, 10 or 20 ml/min. Data were analyzed by analysis of variance. Statistical significance was achieved if $p < 0.05$.

Results

Tobramycin clearances are described in detail in the companion paper [2]. Tobramycin behaved similarly to urea in that its clearance was significantly dependent on both Q_d and UFR. Furthermore, tobramycin appeared to bind to the Biospal AN69 membrane and not to polysulfone membranes.

For each hemofilter the greatest inulin clearance was achieved at a UFR of 20 ml/min. For only two of the five filters studied did this occur at the highest Q_d. Statistically, inulin clearance was independent of Q_d, but highly dependent on UFR. Inulin clearance was greatest in the Biospal at 12.4 ml/min while comparably sized filters had significantly lower inulin clearances (HF500, 9.9 ml/min; D30, 10.1 ml/min). As UFR increased from 0 to 20 ml/min, combined inulin clearance for all filters increased by 355%, while as Q_d increased from 15 to 60 ml/min inulin clearance only rose by 1%.

Table 1. Urea clearances (ml/min)

Filter	Q_d 15 ml/min UFR, ml/min				Q_d 30 ml/min UFR, ml/min				Q_d 60 ml/min UFR, ml/min			
	0	5	10	20	0	5	10	20	0	5	10	20
HF500	11.6	14.3	19.8	29.1	18.5	22.4	25.9	35.7	27.0	24.4	27.2	39.8
Biospal	12.8	16.4	21.0	27.5	18.1	26.6	28.1	34.0	28.0	34.5	34.0	38.7
D30	6.4	16.2	22.2	28.5	15.9	21.5	27.0	36.8	22.7	28.2	29.2	39.7
HF250	8.5	10.6	15.7	22.6	8.7	15.4	20.0	29.8	15.3	17.4	18.1	20.1
D20	8.0	11.0	17.6	21.2	9.0	14.2	18.4	26.9	12.5	13.8	20.1	22.3

Each number is the mean of 6 observations (three filters, and duplication of each combination of flows).

The mean urea clearances for all filters are summarized in table 1. For comparably sized filters there were no differences in urea clearance. Both Q_d and UFR significantly affected urea clearance in each filter. In the absence of ultrafiltration, urea clearances were always less than the Q_d. At maximum UFR, urea clearances among comparably sized filters were equal. For all filters combined, as UFR rose from 0 to 20 ml/min, urea clearance increased by 204% while, as Q_d rose from 15 to 60 ml/min, urea clearance increased by 52%.

Discussion

In patients with catabolic acute renal failure, maximum urea clearance is indicated. In certain related conditions the removal of larger-molecular-weight species may also be beneficial [3]. Thus, maximizing both convection and diffusion is a goal of continuous therapies. However, convectively derived solute removal may lower the concentration gradient for diffusion [2, 4]. On the other hand, we have shown that the presence of dialysate does not affect UFR [5].

The present study demonstrates that inulin clearance is mainly dependent on convection. In contrast, urea clearance is enhanced by increasing either Q_d or UFR. We could not confirm the Sigler and Teehan observation that in CAVHD urea clearance equals Q_d [6]. The combined urea clearance data of the HF500, D30 and Biospal are plotted versus UFR at Q_ds of 15 and 60 ml/min in figure 1. It is clear from this figure that, as UFR increases, small-solute clearance is less dependent on Q_d and when UFR equals plasma flow there is no effect from Q_d.

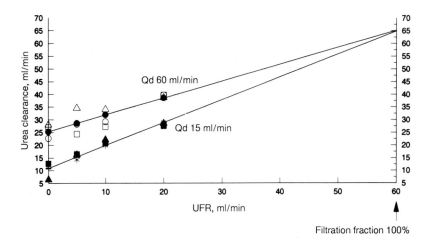

Fig. 1. The urea clearances from the HF500, D30 and Biospal are combined. There is a linear increase in urea clearance for each Q_d as UFR is increased. If projected out at a UFR of 60 ml/min by linear regression analysis, urea clearance at Q_d of 15 ml/min will equal the urea clearance at Q_d 60 ml/min. A UFR of 60 ml/min represents a filtration fraction of 100%.

These results suggest that there are no adverse consequences to maximizing both convection and diffusion. The widest spectrum of molecular weight species will be best removed under these conditions.

References

1   Geronemus R, Schneider N: Continuous arteriovenous hemodialysis: A new modality for treatment of acute renal failure. Trans ASAIO 1984;30:610–612.
2   Cigarran-Guldris S, Brier ME, Golper TA: Tobramycin clearance during simulated continuous arteriovenous hemodialysis; in Sieberth HG, Mann H, Stummvoll HK (eds): Continuous Hemofiltration. Contrib Nephrol. Basel, Karger, 1991, vol 93, pp 120–123.
3   Coraim F, Wolner E: Management of cardiac surgery patients with continuous arteriovenous hemofiltration; in Sieberth HG, Mann H (eds): Continuous Arteriovenous Hemofiltration (CAVH). Basel, Karger, 1985, pp 103–110.
4   Sprenger KGB, Stephan H, Kratz W, Huber K, Franz HE: Optimizing of hemodiafiltration with modern membranes? in Berlyne GH, Giovannetti S (eds): Contr Nephrol. Basel, Karger, 1985, vol 46, pp 43–60.
5   Golper TA, Leone M: Backtransport of dialysate solutes during in vitro continuous arteriovenous hemodialysis. Blood Purif 1989;7:223–229.
6   Sigler MH, Teehan BP: Solute transport in continuous hemodialysis: A new treatment for acute renal failure. Kidney Int 1987;32:562–571.

T.A. Golper, MD, University of Louisville, 500 South Floyd Street,
Louisville, KY 40292 (USA)

Sieberth HG, Mann H, Stummvoll HK (eds): Continuous Hemofiltration.
Contrib Nephrol. Basel, Karger, 1991, vol 93, pp 149–151

Go-Slow Dialysis Instead of Continuous Arteriovenous Hemofiltration

R. Hombrouckx, A.M. Bogaert, F. Leroy, J.Y. De Vos, L. Larno

Dialysis Unit, Kliniek Hogerlucht, Ronse, Belgium

For acute patients in hospitals without a dialysis infrastructure, continuous arteriovenous hemofiltration (CAVH) [1, 2] has proved to be a valuable epuration technique. However, problems of clotting, insufficient ultrafiltration, inadequate clearances in severely catabolic patients limited its use [3]. We tried to combine the advantages of classical dialysis and of the CAVH for treating acute patients. Therefore, we dialyzed the patient with a blood flow of ca. 80 ml/min, by use of a single needle blood pump on a central venous catheter, during ca. 10 h daily in combination with a closed low volume recirculating bicarbonate dialysate.

Materials

The following materials were used: double head pump BL 760 (Bellco, Mirandola, Italy) [4, 5]; recirculating dialysate monitor BL 747 (Bellco) [6]; central catheter: Vas-cath SC 2100 (Gambro) [7, 8]; blood lines: BL 360 (venous) + BL 307 (arterial) (Bellco); artificial kidney: can be of any type.

Methods

An 8-French central catheter is introduced in the subclavian [9], jugular or femoral vein; the patient is dialyzed during ca. 10 h with a blood flow of 80 ml/min using the Bellco double head pump at very low pump head speeds, the ultrafiltration is monitored by the pressure setting in the circuit between the two pump heads, and the dialysate system is a closed recirculating low volume bicarbonate dialysate system of 40 liters, eventually replaced once or twice by fresh dialysate after 3–4 h dialysis (dialysate flow, 500 ml/min).

Discussion

The advantages of 'go-slow dialysis' are that the epuration is softer and more continuous compared to the classical open dialysate high flow hemodialysis: no symptoms of disequilibrium, sudden hypotensions, cramps, nausea, vomiting, etc., occurred. An easy body fluid and electrolyte composition monitoring is possible. Further, blood flow and ultrafiltration are completely independent of the arterial pressure of the patient or eventually of the venous resistance (in case of CAVH on a shunt); also, they are independent of the type of kidney, length and type of blood lines, height of ultrafiltration reservoir, etc.

Ultrafiltration and blood flow are mutually independent because of a separated blood flow setting and ultrafiltration setting possibility; furthermore, by the use of bicarbonate dialysate, there is no risk for lactic acidosis, which can easily occur in severely ill patients with some degree of hypoxemia hypotension, diabetes, liver insufficiency, etc. The low volume dialysate system permits an individualization of the dialysate: there is the possibility of adding sodium, potassium, glucose, oxygen, etc. to the dialysate, also of heparin, which results in an extremely low systematic heparinization with less bleeding tendency in the patient.

Like CAVH, go-slow dialysis rarely provokes, in contrast to the classical short dialysis, stress ulcers in acute patients. As for CAVH, an intravenous hyperalimentation is made possible. There are relatively low risks of thrombosis in the blood circuit and the vessels; no regular flushing of the artificial kidney is needed, and in contrast to CAVH, the solute removal and the clearance ratios are sufficiently high even for highly catabolic patients.

Complementary advanges over CAVH are that no surgery is needed, there is no waste of time in the actue phase as only one catheter is needed, and that this catheter is placed intravenously and not intra-arterially, without risk for bleeding, vascular defect or arterial thrombosis. The patients are less immobilized than in CAVH, and there are less infectious complications of vascular access site. Any type of artificial kidney can be used, not necessarily biocompatible membranes; there is an easy temperature control during the epuration and the costs are less than for CAVH. On the other hand, a nephrologist and a dialysis infrastructure are required but the specialized (trained) paramedical staff has only to intervene in order to start and end the dialysis, and once or twice for changing the dialysate tank. In between the patient is monitored by automatic blood pressure measuring and heart monitoring, under control of the nurses of the intensive care unit.

The normal therapeutic measurements continue during the go-slow dialysis. Occasionally there is a dialysis alarm (for example when changing a patient's position), and at that moment the intensive care nurses warn the dialysis nurses for correcting the deficient parameter (this only occurs once or twice daily).

Conclusion

The advantages of the continuous method of treatment, that is CAVH, are combined with the advantages of a single needle dialysis system, which makes the epuration technique quite independent from parameters such as the patient's arterial pressure, venous resistance, arterial blood flow, etc. Blood flow (in order to obtain a certain clearance) and ultrafiltration (pressure in the blood compartment of the artifical kidney in order to obtain a certain ultrafiltration rate) can be regulated totally independently of each other. An impregnation of the membrane by heparin through the dialysate side allows a very low systematic anticoagulation. The use of bicarbonate is superior to that of lactate especially in acutely ill patients. Unfortunately a dialysis infrastructure is needed, but once installed, the interventions of the dialysis nurse are minimal.

References

1   Kramer P, Wigger W, Rieger J, Matthaei D, Scheler F: Arteriovenous hemofiltration: A new and simple method for treatment of overhydrated patients resistant to diuretics. Klin Wochenschr 1977;55:1121.
2   Juan P, Bosch JP, Ronco C: Continuous arteriovenous hemofiltration in Maher S (ed): Replacement of Renal Function by Dialysis, ed 3. New York, Kluwer Academic Publishers, 1989, chap 15, pp 347–354.
3   Kaplan AA: Enhanced efficiency during CAVH: La Greca G, Fabris A, Ronco C (eds): Clinical Trials with Predilution and Vacuum Suction in CAVH. Milan, Wichtig, 1986, p 49.
4   Van Waeleghem JP, Boone L. Ringoir S: New technique on the one needle system during haemodialysis. Eur Dial Transplant Nurses Assoc 1973;1:10.
5   De Vos JY, Van Wetter Ph, De Rekeneire G, Vanderbeken M, Larno L, Hombrouckx R: Introduction of an arterial expansion chamber (AEC) using a low compliance artificial kidney on the double head pump (DHP). Single Needle Dialysis Monogram EDTNA-ERCA, pp 17–22.
6   De Vos JY, Larno L, De Rekeneire G, Leroy F, Hombrouckx R: Acute dialysis: Advantages of a low volume closed recirculating bicarbonate dialysate system. EDTNA, Madrid 1982, p 46.
7   Shaldon S, Chiandussi L, Higgs B: Haemodialysis by percutaneous catheterisation of the femoral artery and vein with regional heparinisation. Lancet 1961;ii:857.
8   Bambauer R, Jutzler GA: Erfahrungen mit grosslumigen Verweilkathetern in der V. jugularis interna als Zugang für akute Hämodialysen. Klin Wocheschr 1982;60:285.
9   Quinton WE, Dillard D, Scribner BH: Cannulation of blood vessels for prolonged hemodialysis. Trans Am Soc Artif Intern Organs 1960;6:104.

R. Hombrouckx, MD, Dialysis Unit, Kliniek Hogerlucht, Hogerluchtstraat 6, B–9600 Ronse (Belgium)

Sieberth, HG, Mann H, Stummvoll HK (eds): Continuous Hemofiltration.
Contrib Nephrol. Basel, Karger, 1991, vol 93, pp 152–155

Lactate or Bicarbonate for Intermittent Hemofiltration?

*M. Clasen, R. Böhm, J. Riehl, U. Gladziwa, K.V. Dakshinamurty,
B. Schacht, H. Mann, H.G. Sieberth*

Department of Internal Medicine II, Technical University of Aachen, FRG

Continuous hemofiltration (HF) has been widely accepted as a therapy
for acute renal failure specially in critically ill patients with multiple organ
failure. Continuous HF has 3 aims: (1) detoxification of blood; (2) removal
of fluid overload; and (3) compensation of metabolic acidosis.

For the latter aim, commercial substitution fluids for intermittent HF
contain 30–45 mmol/1 lactate. However, lactate is thought to have negative effects on metabolic and hemodynamic parameters. In our clinic we
observed several times lactic acidosis during lactate-buffered HF (LBHF)
in some patients, which gave the reason for the present study.

Bicarbonate-buffered substitution fluids are commercially not available
because readily mixed fluids containing bicarbonate are not stable for days.
As an alternative we used buffer-free solutions which were mixed with
bicarbonate immediately before use. The aim of our study was to compare
the effects of bicarbonate- and lactate-buffered HF substitution fluids in
patients with chronic renal insufficiency undergoing intermittent HF.

Patients and Methods

The intraindividual changes in metabolic and hemodynamic parameters in 11 patients
undergoing chronic intermittent HF were evaluated in a 9-week crossover trial comparing
bicarbonate-buffered HF (BBHF) with LBHF (fig. 1). The patients underwent intermittent
HF at regular intervals 3 times a week. The demographic data are given in table 1. The
following parameters were controlled at the beginning, during and at the end of each HF: pH;
standard bicarbonate; base excess; blood glucose; plasma lactate (Enzymatic test, DuPont;
sodium-fluoride-containing test tubes); potassium; heart rate, and systolic, diastolic and mean
arterial blood pressure. The 2 different lactate-buffered solution fluids used in the trial
contained: sodium, 138 or 142 mmol/l; potassium, 0 or 2 mmol/l; calcium, 2 mmol/l; magnesium, 0.75 mmol/l; chloride, 103 or 111.5 mmol/l; lactate, 34 or 44.5 mmol/l, and glucose,
0 mmol/l. The bicarbonate solution fluids contained: sodium, 105 mmol/l; potassium, 0 or
2 mmol/l; calcium, 1.75 mmol/l; magnesium, 0.5 mmol/l; chloride, 109.5 mmol/l; lactate,
3 mmol/l; glucose, 1 gl/l, and bicarbonate, 34.4 mmol/l. LBHF and BBHF periods were
identical as concerns the duration of treatment, amounts of substitute and net ultrafiltration.
Statistical analysis was performed by analysis of variance and paired Student's *t* test.

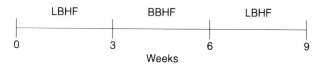

Fig. 1. Study protocol of the 9-week crossover trial. Solution fluids contained in **LBHF** 44.5 mmol/l lactate and in **BBHF** 34.4 mmol/l bicarbonate and 3 mmol/l lactate.

Table 1. Patient data

Female/male ratio	4/7
Age, years	
Mean	61.6
Range	51–76
Duration of HF treatment, months	
Mean	35
Range	1–98
Diagnoses	
Hypertension	7
Chronic pyelonephritis	4
Diabetes mellitus	3
Chronic glomerulonephritis	1
Goodpasture's syndrome	1
Malignant hypertension	1
Multiple myeloma	1

Results

LBHF increased mean plasma lactate levels in all patients from basal 1.37 ± 0.9 to 6.4 ± 2.1 mmol/l at the end of HF (normal range < 2.6 mmol/l). All 3 diabetic patients in our study group developed the highest lactate levels which rose to > 10 mmol/l. In contrast, BBHF led to significantly ($p < 0.001$) lower basal lactate levels (0.95 ± 0.4 mmol/l) followed by a slight increase to 1.1 ± 0.4 mmol/l.

Surprisingly, all parameters of acid-base balance (mean pH levels, standard bicarbonate, base excess) showed a better control of metabolic acidosis by LBHF than by BBHF (table 2). Standard bicarbonate levels raised more slowly during LBHF than during BBHF with no change during the first part of the treatment. Nevertheless, at the end of HF, mean standard bicarbonate levels were significantly higher ($p < 0.001$) during LBHF.

Blood glucose and potassium levels were similar during both treatments. Mean arterial blood pressure, heart rate and the number of hy-

Table 2. Mean values of pH and standard bicarbonate (mmol/1)

Time of HF	LBHF		BBHF		LBHF	
	pH	bicarbonate	pH	bicarbonate	pH	bicarbonate
Before	7.34	19.4	7.30*	16.6*	7.36	19.7
During	7.39	19.5	7.35*	18.2*	7.40	20.2
End	7.42	21.6	7.37*	18.7*	7.43	22.3

* $p < 0.005$.

potensive periods were comparable during **LBHF** and **BBHF**, showing no statistically significant difference.

A questionnaire about subjective feelings given to the patients showed that 3 out of 11 patients felt subjectively better during the bicarbonate treatment. Especially, scores for pruritus tended to be lower under this treatment, whereas complaints of headache and nausea were unchanged.

Discussion

Lactate as a buffer precursor must be metabolized to bicarbonate to achieve compensation of metabolic acidosis. The high values of plasma lactate found are well known from patients with severe lactic acidosis. In case of impaired liver function, sepsis or hypoxemia, lactate can accumulate in critically ill patients and metabolic acidosis will be additionally intensified [1]. A renal replacement therapy for patients with multiorgan failure must consider this undesired side effect. Nevertheless, no lactic acidosis was found during this chronic intermittent therapy. Bicarbonate as the physiological buffer has been widely established for acute hemodialysis [2]. For reasons like chemical instability, the readily mixed bicarbonate-containing substitution fluids are not available for HF. We could demonstrate in the present study that a buffer-free solution which is mixed with bicarbonate immediately before use is a practical and safe alternative. Buffering effects of bicarbonate could be proven directly after the start of HF, whereas LBHF increases standard bicarbonate not before 2 h of treatment. The overall better buffering effect of LBHF in our study is not related to the presence of lactate or bicarbonate in the substitution fluid, but to the higher quantity of buffer. In contrast to other authors [3], we suggest that bicarbonate concentrations should contain about 40 mmol/1 to produce a sufficient buffering effect. In general, buffer concentrations should be adapted to the individual requirement of the patients which can be estimated by the daily urea generation rate [4].

It is clear that bicarbonate is the buffer of choice for acute renal replacement therapy even if its applicability for chronic and intermittent HF seems to be more difficult.

In conclusion: (1) lactate as a buffer equivalent in intermittent HF increases plasma lactate levels far above the normal range; (2) but lactate for intermittent HF produces better control of metabolic acidosis compared to bicarbonate buffer (34.4 mmol/l); (3) BBHF is a safe and practical alternative to LBHF, especially for continuous treatment in critically ill patients prone to lactic acidosis, and (4) for intermittent HF, the bicarbonate concentration of substitution fluids should be higher than 35 mmol/l.

References

1   Mizock BA: Controversies in lactic acidosis. JAMA 1987;258:497–501.
2   Leunissen KML, van Hoof JP: Acetate or bicarbonate for hemodialysis? Nephrol Dial Transplant 1988;3:1–7.
3   Vlaho M: Bikarbonat-Hämofiltration versus Laktat-Hämofiltration. Nieren- Hochdruckkrankheiten 1990;7:285–290.
4   Stiller S, Mann H: Comparison of different methods of blood detoxification; in Sieberth HG, Mann H: Continuous Arteriovenous Hemofiltration (CAVH). Basel, Karger, 1985, pp 143–151.

Dr. Wolfgang Clasen, Krankenhaus der Missionsschwestern Hiltrup,
Westfalenstrasse 109, D–W–4400 Münster (FRG)

Sieberth HG, Mann H, Stummvoll HK (eds): Continuous Hemofiltration.
Contrib Nephrol. Basel, Karger, 1991, vol 93, pp 156–161

Continuous Arteriovenous Hemofiltration Improvement by Adding Diffusion and Adsorption

R. Marangoni, F. Civardi, R. Savino, F. Masi

Nephrology and Dialysis Unit, Bollate, Italy

Continuous arteriovenous hemofiltration (CAVH) may not be efficient enough for the treatment of hypercatabolic uremic patients because of its low ultrafiltration rate (UFR) and consequently of its low efficiency per unit of time. Aiming at improving CAVH performances, some modifications to the standard method were performed: (a) application of negative pressure on the ultrafiltrate line [1]; (b) use of predilution on the arterial line [2]; (c) insertion of a blood pump on the arterial line [3]; (d) use of hemofilters with larger surface [4]; (e) combination of diffusion and convection by infusion of dialysate into the ultrafiltrate compartment of the hemofilter: continuously with low flow rate (continuous arteriovenous hemodialysis: CAVHD) [5] or periodically with high flow rate (arteriovenous hemodiafiltration: AVHDF) [6]. According to our findings the insertion of a cartridge containing collodion-coated activated charcoal (CAC) microencapsulated in the extracorporeal circuit can remarkably improve the efficiency of the convective blood purification methods either with pump-assisted (hemofiltration: HF) [7] or with spontaneous extra-corporeal circulation (CAVH) [8]. The addition of hemoperfusion (HP) remarkably increases the removal of creatinine, uric acid, guanidines, phenols, middle molecules, PTH, β_2-microglobulin; it increases urea removal negligibly; the adsorbent does not remove water, electrolytes, organic acids and phosphate [8, 9]. HP addition to convective methods remarkably increases the clearances of many but not of all the uremic toxins. On the contrary, AVHDF through the added diffusion gives a lower but more general increase of the clearances especially of those of small molecules [10]. Therefore, we built an extracorporeal circuit in which, after the hemofilter arranged for AVHDF, we inserted a cartridge containing CAC, performing so CAVH + HP treatments alternating with AVHDF + HP ones (fig. 1). The last combination was performed with the purpose of

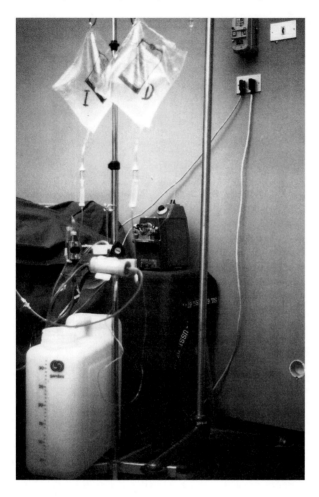

Fig. 1. Working AVHDF + HP.

carrying out a blood purification method as efficiently as possible with extracorporeal spontaneous circulation and with the same high tolerability of the standard CAVH.

Materials and Methods

In a usual extracorporeal circuit for CAVH, after the hemofilter (Amicon D20, surface $0.25\,m^2$, polysulfone) we inserted a cartridge containing 70 g of CAC microencapsulated (Sorbex 70). The cartridge venous port is connected to a drip-chamber which goes on the venous set where the reinfusion point (postdilutional method) is. The ultrafiltrate compartment of the hemofilter has two accesses: one for dialysate inlet, another for dialysate and

Table 1. Population baseline data

	Patient					
	1	2	3	4	5	6
Age, years	28	57	66	4	61	58
Sex	m	f	m	f	f	m
Diagnosis (post surgical)	ARF	ARF	ARF	ARF	ARF	ARF
Dry body weight, kg	74	79	81	84	78	70
Fluid overload, kg	2.5	3.0	3.5	2.0	1.5	3.5
Vascular access[1]						
Qb, ml/min	80	100	120	90	80	110

Session number: 3 according to protocol A, alternating with 3 according to protocol B.
[1]Quinton-Scribner shunt.

ultrafiltrate outlet. The solution employed either as reinfusion fluid or as dialysate is normal replacement solution for HF. The system washing is performed by the infusion of 3,000 ml of heparinized saline solution (2,500 IU/l) preheated at 37 °C. During the treatment, heparinized solution is infused into the arterial line in such a way to maintain the coagulation time at 15–20 min (Lee-White) for determinations made on the venous line.

We carried out 2 different treatment protocols:

Protocol A: (1) CAVH + HP for the first 6 h; (2) CAVH for the rest of the time: 18 h; (whole session time: 24 h).

Protocol B: (1) AVHDF (infusion of dialysate by gravity into the ultrafiltrate compartment of the hemofilter: 300 ml/min) for the first 3 h; (2) CAVH + HP for the next 3 h; (3) CAVH for the rest of the time: 18 h (whole session time: 24 h).

Our whole population of treated patients consists of 6 cases (table 1) affected by acute renal failure with anuria, for whom the standard CAVH was not efficient enough because of superimposed severe catabolic states due to septic episodes. Each patient underwent 3 treatments according to protocol A alternating with 3 treatments performed according to protocol B.

During the treatments the following were determined: (a) urea, creatinine, uric acid, guanidine clearances in CAVH or AVHDF section and in whole system (CAVH + HP or AVHDF + HP) at different times; (b) percentage decrease of urea, creatinine, uric acid, guanidine serum levels during treatment performed according to two protocols; (c) platelet and leukocyte number; (d) blood flow in the extracorporeal circuit with and without Sorbex 70 aiming at verifying possible variation due to the cartridge insertion.

Results

The results obtained show (table 2) that HP addition negligibly increases urea clearance, while it remarkably increases creatinine, uric acid, guanidine clearances. The highest performances are obtained with the combination AVHDF + HP. The satisfactory efficiency of Sorbex 70 goes on until the 6th hour; after this time the cartridge must be removed (easy

Table 2. Clearances (ml/min) due to CAVH, AVHDF sections and to combined systems (CAVH + HP, AVHDF + HP)

Time		Urea	Creatinine	Uric acid	Guanidine
15 min	CAVH	10	10	7	6
	AVHDF	26	27	26	21
	CAVH + HP	12	51	70	65
	AVHDF + HP	27	68	95	84
135 min	CAVH	10	10	7	6
	AVHDF	26	27	25	20
	CAVH + HP	12	52	70	65
	AVHDF + HP	27	64	95	83
180 min	CAVH	10	10	7	6
	AVHDF	25	26	25	20
	CAVH + HP	11	51	70	65
	AVHDF + HP	27	62	95	83
255 min	CAVH	10	10	7	6
	CAVH + HP	11	50	70	65
360 min	CAVH	10	9	6	5
	CAVH + HP	11	48	66	59
375 min	CAVH	10	9	6	6
24 h	CAVH	9	7	5	5

Qb 120 ml/min; Ht 28%.

operation). Figures 2 and 3 show the percentage decrease of urea, creatinine, uric acid, guanidine serum levels during sessions according to two protocols. The different serum level lowering of the considered molecules confirms the clearance trend: HP addition remarkably increases creatinine, uric acid, guanidine removal, but negligibly the urea one. AVHDF almost uniformly increases the removal of the 4 uremic toxins. Sorbex 70 insertion causes a low increase of the resistances and consequently a low decrease (5%) of the blood flow in the extracorporeal circuit (fig. 4).

The method proved to be well tolerated. We did not notice shivers, fever, bodily discomfort, significantly modifications of heart rate and mean arterial pressure. The heparin dose is the same which is necessary for standard CAVH. The platelet and leukocyte number did not show modifications more evident than those noticed in the standard method.

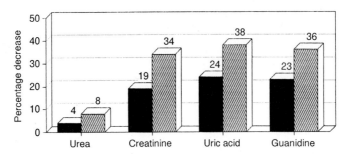

Fig. 2. Percentage decrease of urea, creatinine, uric acid, guanidine serum levels during treatment according to protocol A. ■ = Third hour; ▨ = sixth hour. Mean of 3 determinations in the same patient (Qb 120 ml/min; Ht 28%).

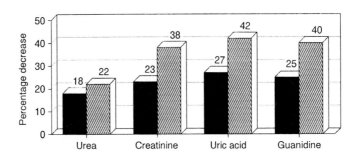

Fig. 3. Percentage decrease of urea, creatinine, uric acid, guanidine serum levels during treatment according to protocol B. ■ = Third hour; ▨ = sixth hour. Mean of 3 determinations in the same patient (Qb 120 ml/min; Ht 28%).

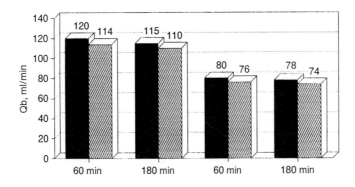

Fig. 4. Blood flow change by adding Sorbex 70 at 60 and 180 min. ■ = CAVH only; ▨ = CAVH + HP.

Discussion

According to our experience the addition of HP to CAVH and to AVHDF deserves a place among the modifications of the standard CAVH aiming at improving its efficiency. It is true that not all uremic toxins are removed with the same rate. But we must consider: (a) among the molecules highly removed by HP there are very important uremic toxins; (b) the combination AVHDF + HP however causes a whole increase of the uremic toxins removal.

In fact, the addition of diffusion and adsorption to CAVH gives the highest performances achievable by a blood purification method with spontaneous extracorporeal circulation. That gives us the possibility of treating hypercatabolic uremic patients with serious cardiovascular instability with a highly efficient method which shows the same tolerability of the standard CAVH.

References

1   Kaplan AA, Longnecker RE, Folkert VW: Suction-assisted continuous arteriovenous hemofiltration. Trans Am Soc Artif Intern Organs 1983;29:408–412.
2   Williams V, Perkins L: Continuous ultrafiltration. A new ICU procedure for the treatment of fluid overload. Crit Care Nursing Q 1984;4:4–44.
3   Kaplan AA: The effect of predilution during continuous arteriovenous hemofiltration (abstract). Am Soc Nephrol 1984;17:66A.
4   Lysaght MJ, Schmidt B, Gurland HJ: Filtration rates and pressure driving forces in AV filtration. An experimental study. Blood Purif 1983;1:178–183.
5   Geronemus R, Schneider N: Continuous arteriovenous hemodialysis: A new modality for treatment of acute renal failure. Trans Am Soc Artif Intern Organs 1984;30:610–613.
6   Ronco C, Brendolan A, Bragantini L, Chiaramonte S, Fabris A, Feriani M, Dell'Aquila R, Milan M, La Greca G: Arteriovenous hemodiafiltration associated with continuous arteriovenous hemofiltration: A combined therapy for acute renal failure in the hypercatabolic patient. Blood Purif 1987;5:33–40.
7   Marangoni R, Civardi F, Masi F, Avanzi C, Savino R, Manfredi A: Continuous arteriovenous hemofiltration (CAVH) combined with hemoperfusion (HP) Proc Int Symp on Continuous Arteriovenous Hemofiltration, Vicenza, April 1986, pp 111–116.
8   Marangoni R, Civardi F, Savino R, Manfredi A, Avanzi C, Masi F, Cimino R, Colombo R: Hemofiltration (HF) efficiency improvement by adding hemoperfusion (HP). Abstr VIIth ISAO, Sapporo, 1989, p 331.
9   Gelfand MC: Hemoperfusion in uremia at the crossroads: Is there a true role? 8th Int Congr Nephrol, Athens, 1981, p 400.
10 Marangoni R, Civardi F: Continuous arteriovenous hemofiltration combined with arteriovenous hemodiafiltration and hemoperfusion (abstract). Blood Purif 1986;4:221.

Roberto Marangoni, MD, Bollate Hospital, Via Piave 20, I–20021 Bollate-MI (Italy)

Sieberth HG, Mann H, Stummvoll HK (eds): Continuous Hemofiltration.
Contrib Nephrol. Basel, Karger, 1991, vol 93, pp 162–166

Filtration Rate and Sieving Coefficients of Six Different Filters for Continuous Hemofiltration

W.M. Glöckner, M. Gerarts

Medical Clinic II, RWTH Aachen, FRG

Within the last decade continuous arteriovenous (CAVH) and pump-assisted venovenous hemofiltration (CVVH) have become established for patients suffering from acute renal failure (ARF) [1–3]. For optimal treatment a comparison of commercially available filter modules with regard to filtration flow and sieving curve is desirable. We therefore analysed ex vivo filtration rate, transmembrane pressure and sieving coefficients of six different hemofilters in each of a group of 6 patients.

Materials and Methods

The analyzed six hemofilters with their module and membrane characteristics are listed in table 1.

After rinsing with 3 liters of physiological saline, adding 5,000 U of heparin into the last liter, the filter was fit in the extracorporeal circuit maintained by a roller blood pump and a double-lumen catheter inserted in the vena jugularis interna or the vena subclavia. Increasing the blood flow stepwise the filtration flow and pressure measurements before and behind the filter were done. After 1 h blood and filtrate samples were collected for the measurement of sieving coefficients defined by the ratio of concentration in filtrate/plasma. Thus, all the six hemofilters could be analyzed one after the other in one session.

Creatinine was measured by the Jaffé reaction with the creatinine analyzer 2 from Beckman, β_2-microglobulin by radioimmunoassay (Beta$_2$-micro Ria 100) from Pharmacia. The analysis of retinol-binding protein, acidic α_1-glycoprotein and prealbumin was done with the laser-nephelometer from Behring.

Results

In a retrospective analysis of 26 patients with ARF we examined the running duration of the hemofilter AV 600, we could not find a dependance from the hematocrit, the dosage of heparin (between 200 and 1,500 U/h) or the activated clotting time (between 100 and 170 s). The average running time was 44.4 h with a range from 5.8 to 97.0 h.

The six hemofilters analyzed differ substantially in filtration rate shown in figures 1–3: with a constant blood flow of 100 ml/min filtrate flow

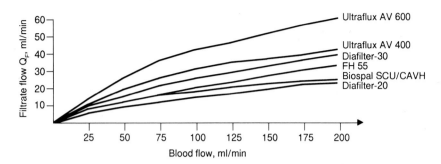

Fig. 1. Filtrate flow Q_F in relation to blood flow for six different hemofilters (number of patients = 6).

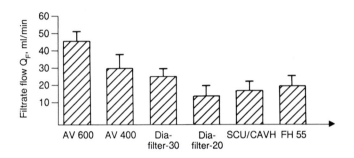

Fig. 2. Filtrate flow Q_F ($\pm$SD) with a fixed blood flow of 100 ml/min (n = 6).

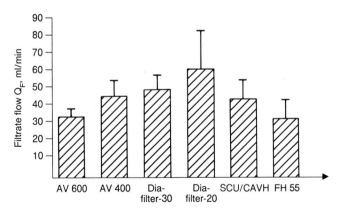

Fig. 3. Filtrate flow Q_F ($\pm$SD) with a blood flow of 100 ml/min normalized for a membrane surface area of 1.0 m^2 (n = 6).

Table 1. Data of the analyzed hemofilters (following the instructions of the producer)

	Producer	Type of filter	Membrane type	Effective membrane surface m²	Filling volume ml	Cut-off dalton
Ultraflux AV 600	Fresenius	capillary filter	polysulfone	1.35	90	
Ultraflux AV 400	Fresenius	capillary filter	polysulfone	0.70	48	
Dialfilter-30	Amicon	capillary filter	polysulfone	0.55	40	50,000
Dialfilter-20	Amicon	capillary filter	polysulfone	0.25	27	50,000
Biospal SCU/CAVH	Hospal	flat membrane filter	polyacrylonitrile	0.50	60	40,000
Fiber Hemofilter FH55	Gambro	capillary filter	polyamide	0.60	43	25,000

Table 2. Mean sieving coefficients of 6 hemofilters ($\pm$ SD)

Marker molecule	Molecular weight dalton	Biospal SCU/CAVH (Hospal)	Ultraflux AV 600 (Fresenius)	Ultraflux AV 400 (Fresenius)	Fiber hemofilter FH55 (Gambro)	Diafilter-30 hemofilter (Amicon)	Diafilter-20 hemofilter (Amicon)
Creatinine	113	0.984 ±0.074	0.991 ±0.095	0.979 ±0.110	0.978 ±0.069	1.030 ±0.062	1.017 ±0.086
β_2-Microglobulin	11,818	0.382 ±0.147	0.311 ±0.160	0.306 ±0.056	0.067 ±0.011	0.033 ±0.058	0.004 ±0.008
Retinol-binding protein	21,000	0.027 ±0.025	0.003 ±0.005	0.004 ±0.005	0.004 ±0.007	—	—

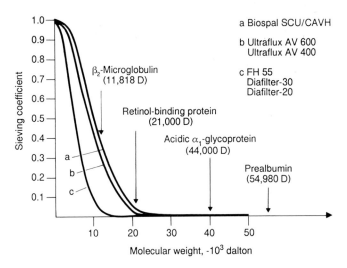

Fig. 4. Sieving coefficients of six hemofilters for molecules of different molecular weight (n = 7).

(Q_F) ranges from 16 to 47 ml/min and with a constant plasma flow of 100 ml/min Q_F ranges from 22 to 65 ml/min.

There is no linear relationship between blood flow and filtrate flow (fig. 1). Depending on the membrane surface area there is a tendency to a filtration plateau, which is not yet reached even for the smallest filters with a blood flow of 200 ml/min.

The highest filtration rate is found in the filter with the largest membrane surface (fig. 2), but in relation to the surface area the smaller filters show a relatively higher filtrate flow (fig. 3). With increasing blood flow the transmembrane pressure (TMP) rises linearly with no significant differences between the hemofilters analyzed.

For the membrane permeability we could find major differences: whereas for the small molecules like creatinine the elimination was equally high for all the membranes, the sieving coefficient (SC) for β_2-microglobulin (11.8 kD) was determined between 0.03 and 0.38 for the different hemofilters, and for the retinol-binding protein (21.0 kD) between 0.0 and 0.03. But for all the bigger molecules like the acidic α_1-glycoprotein (44.0 kD) and prealbumin (55.0 kD) the SC was <0.01 for all the membranes, thus no elimination could be found (table 2; fig. 4).

Discussion

The relation of filtrate to blood flow in hemofiltration is not linear: after a linear range of TMP-dependent filtration, the increase of hemofiltrate diminishes due to hemoconcentration inside the filter [4]. Thus, we found that besides from the blood flow the filteration rate depends on the membrane surface area and filter type. Under ex vivo conditions, the polysulfone capillary filter AV 600 showed the highest filtrate flow of the six analyzed hemofilters.

The analysis of the sieving characteristics after a running duration of 1 h demonstrated remarkable elimination of β_2-microglobulin by the PAN flat membrane SCU/CAVH and the AV 600, whereas bigger molecules like retinol-binding protein, acidic α_1-glycoprotein and prealbumin are almost completely retained by all membranes. These data prove that the cut-off values measured in vitro by the manufacturer (table 1) are not comparable to the sieving coefficient curves determined ex vivo.

References

1   Kramer P (ed): Arterio-venöse Hämofiltration-Nieren-(Ersatz)-Therapie im Intensivpflegebereich. Göttingen, Vandenhoeck & Ruprecht, 1982.

2   Sieberth HG, Mann H (ed): Continuous Arterio-Venous Hemofiltration (CAVH). Basel, Karger, 1985.

3   Glöckner WM: Kontinuierliche Hämofiltration – eine praxisbezogene Einführung. Aktuel Nephrol 1986;19:141–150.

4   Göhl H, Konstantin P: Membranes and filters for hemofiltration; in Henderson LW, Quellhorst EA, Baldamus LA, Lysaght MJ (eds): Hemofiltration. Berlin, Springer, 1986, pp 42–82.

Prof. Dr. W.M. Glöckner, Medizinische Klinik II der RWTH, Pauwelsstrasse 30, D–W–5100 Aachen (FRG)

Sieberth HG, Mann H, Stummvoll HK (eds): Continuous Hemofiltration.
Contrib Nephrol. Basel, Karger, 1991, vol 93, pp 167–170

An Automatic System for Fluid Balance in Continuous Hemofiltration with Very High Precision

Wolfgang Heinrichs, Stefan Mönk, Ulrich Fauth, Miklos Halmágyi

Department of Anaesthesiology, Johannes Gutenberg University, Mainz, FRG

There are three problems concerning the fluid balance in hemofiltration. (1) Continuous hemofiltration requires high daily fluid exchange rates from 20 to more than 40 liters. In view of an acceptable error of the daily fluid balance of ± 200 ml, the overall precision of the fluid-balancing system has to be less than 0.5–1%. (2) The rate of the replacement fluid has to be somewhat lower than the actual ultrafiltration rate (e.g. compensation for drug and nutrition solutions and – if present – urine). (3) During the continuous daily treatment the deviation from the dynamic momentary balance has to be less than ± 100 ml.

Methods

We developed an automatic system for the fluid balance (fig. 1) in continuous hemofiltration using 2 electronic balances with RS-232 computer interfaces (Sartorius MP08) for the measurement of the amount of ultrafiltrate and the amount of replacement fluid given, respectively. The system further consists of 2 volumetric pumps (Schiwa 9000) for administration of the replacement fluid (2,000 ml/h maximal rate) and a microprocessor. The software on the microprocessor mainly drives a PID controller with inputs from the user and the balances and output to control the volumetric pumps. The system works automatically and requires only nurse assistance for changing replacement fluid bags or emptying the ultrafiltrate container. A status and error display provides continuous information about the function of the system.

We used the system successfully in 5 patients. The daily fluid exchange rate ranged between 22 and 28 liters (treatment period 3–5 days). We compared the errors of the automatic system to those done by our nurses by recording the momentary deviation from the desired fluid balance using electronic balances.

Results

A typical recording of a manual balancing done by a very well trained nurse is shown in figure 2. We found momentary deviations from the desired level ranging up to 500 ml. The estimated daily error in those cases

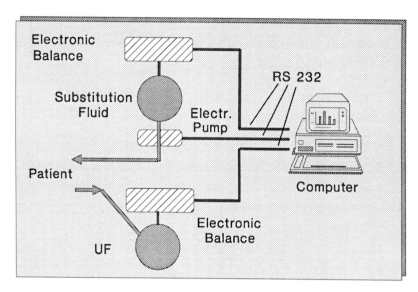

Fig. 1. Schematic drawing of our automatic fluid-balancing system for continuous hemofiltration.

was between 200 ml and more than 1 liter. In contrast, figure 3 shows a recording taken from the automatic system. The momentary deviation is clearly less than 25 ml; in all cases the resulting daily error was found to be less than 20 ml. Thus, the precision of our system is approximately 10 times higher than required.

Discussion

Various methods for fluid balance in hemofiltration include: (1) manual balancing using hourly ultrafiltrate control, this is the classical method suggested by Kramer; (2) manual balancing using electronic balances; (3) automatic balancing with a mechanical device [1]; (4) automatic balancing with an electronic device [2], and (5) automatic balancing using 2 volumetric pumps [3].

There are well-defined problems and pitfalls with these methods. (1) Manual balancing is either extremely time-consuming or of little accuracy. (2) Both the mechanical balance [1] and the electronic balance [2] use a gravity-driven replacement system. In case of pump-assisted continuous venovenous hemofiltration, the pressure generated by the blood pump may interact with the system. Furthermore, as concerns the mechanical system [1], it is difficult to believe that such a system maintains the required precision in daily practice. (3) Volumetric pumps are subject to errors in

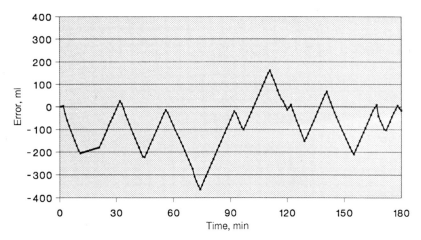

Fig. 2. Recording of the momentary deviation ('error') during manual balancing done by a trained nurse. The maximal deviation is ∼400 ml.

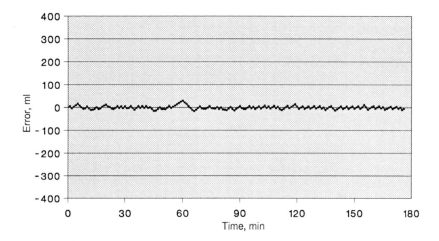

Fig. 3. Recording of the momentary deviation ('error') during automatic balancing with our system. The maximal error is less than 25 ml.

the range of 3–5% [4, 5]. Therefore, the 2- pump system [3] may be less accurate than required.

In contrast, our system has a very high accuracy that was found to be 10 times higher than required. This accuracy is maintained independently from the precision of the pumps. An industrial system could use a very simple roller pump instead of the volumetric pumps. We designed an active system that can be used in any kind of hemofiltration. Finally, our system saves nursing time. Interaction is required in an amount comparable of supervising a volumetric pump. Error detection and alarms are an integral part of the software, and a status profile of the momentary and cumulated fluid balance is continuously provided.

References

1 Schurek HJ, Biela JD, Bergmann KH: Further improvement of a mechanical device for automatic fluid balance in CAVH; in Sieberth HG, Mann H (eds): Continuous Arteriovenous Hemofiltration (CAVH). Basel, Karger, 1985, pp 67–75.

2 Schultheis R, Brings W, Glöckner WM, Sieberth HG: Device for controlled cyclic substitution during spontaneous filtration; in Sieberth HG, Mann H (eds): Continuous Arteriovenous Hemofiltration (CAVH). Basel, Karger, 1985, pp 64–66.

3 Stein B, Maucher H, Wiedeck H, Born B, Ahnefeld FW: Die Steuerung der Ultrafiltrationsrate als Hauptkomponente eines neuen Bilanzierungssystems während kontinuierlicher Hämofiltration. Anaesthesist 1989;38:536–538.

4 Stull JC, Erenberg A, Leff RD: Flow rate variability from electronic infusion devices. Crit Care Med 1988;16:888–891.

5 Stull JC, Schneider PJ, Erenberg A, Leff RD: Decreased flow accuracy from volumetric infusion pumps. Crit Care Med 1989;17:926–928.

Dr. W. Heinrichs, Klinik für Anästhesiologie, Langenbeckstrasse 1,
D–W–6500 Mainz (FRG)

Sieberth HG, Mann H, Stummvoll HK (eds): Continuous Hemofiltration.
Contrib Nephrol. Basel, Karger, 1991, vol 93, pp 171–174

Effects of Access Catheter Dimensions on Bloodflow in Continuous Arteriovenous Hemofiltration[1]

Randall Jenkins[a], *James Funk*[b], *Baoding Chen*[b], *Dirk Thacker*[a]

[a]Department of Pediatrics, University of Louisville, Ky.; [b]Department of Mechanical Engineering, University of Kentucky, Ky., USA

Numerous catheters have been introduced commercially for use in CAVH systems; however, most data on flow in CAVH systems are given using either Scribner shunts, Vygon 3-mm catheters, or catheters of unspecified length [1–3]. Therefore, little is known concerning the effect of catheter dimension on CAVH bloodflow. We hypothesize the CAVH bloodflow can be predicted as a function of catheter dimensions for specified CAVH systems. This is accomplished with a combined experimental and theoretical approach for three commercial CAVH systems.

Methods

Flow of distilled water was measured in a CAVH system operated with an in vitro apparatus which allows accurate setting of various pressure heads. Use of a similar apparatus has previously been reported [4]. Flow was measured with graduated cylinder and stopwatch. The system was an Amicon (Amicon Corp., Danvers, Mass.) D3O® (new) CAVH system. The system included a hemofilter, arterial and venous tubing, and two 7-Fr Medcomp 4.5-inch catheters (Medical Components, Inc., Harleysville, Pa.).

Flow characteristics of the Medcomp CAVH catheters and a set of Amicon CAVH tubings were determined using the above-mentioned apparatus. The method for determination of flow characteristics was previously published [5]. Each device is uniquely described by a set of three flow characteristics, D, L and K, where D is the inner diameter, L is the length of the narrow bore portion of the device, and K is a factor which accounts for changes in diameter and entrance and exit losses.

A computer simulation of CAVH bloodflow has previously been developed and tested [5]. Given an input of driving pressures, catheter and tubing flow characteristics, hemofilter end-to-end pressure drop data, hematocrit, temperature, and protein concentration, the CAVH bloodflow and pressure distribution can be predicted.

Computer simulations were performed for the CAVH system described above. Input into the simulations were the same conditions as were found for the distilled water

[1] This work was supported by a grant from the Alliant Community Trust.

Table 1. Experiments and predicted CAVH system flow for distilled water at 25 °C: Amicon D30 CAVH system flow (ml/min)

Actual	Predicted	Difference %
43.5	46.4	6.6
56.4	57.4	1.7
77.5	76.9	0.8
95.6	94.7	0.9
105.0	103.9	1.0

experiments. End-to-end pressure drop data for the hemofilters used for these simulations were obtained by experiment. The results of the simulations were compared to experimental results.

Finally, computer simulations for three commercial CAVH systems were performed with conditions chosen which might occur clinically. Systems were chosen to represent the spectrum of CAVH hemofilter resistance. Bloodflow was predicted for catheters of various dimensions. Input mean arterial and venous pressures were selected to be 70 and 15 mm Hg, respectively. The blood hematocrit and total protein concentrations were chosen to be 30 and 6.5 g/dl, respectively. End-to-end flow resistance was determined from the manufacturer's data, or by experiment with fluid of known viscosity.

Results

Flow characteristics for the Medcomp CAVH catheters and 2 tubings were obtained. Correlations of data points to predicted curves of pressure versus flow were good (>95%) in all cases.

Actual and predicted flow of distilled water through an Amicon CAVH system are shown in table 1. The mean error of flow prediction is 2%.

Figure 1 shows predictions of bloodflow under presumed clinically applicable conditions (pressures and blood characteristics) for 3 low flow resistance *(a)*, average flow resistance, *(b)*, and high flow resistance *(c)* systems. These predictions are depicted for catheter inner diameter varying up to 4.0 mm. A rapid increase in bloodflow is predicted as ID increases from 0 to approximately 2.0 mm. As catheter ID increases above 2.0 mm, system bloodflow increases but appears to approach a plateau. Bloodflow through system *(a)* plateaus at levels more than twice that through system *(c)*.

Bloodflows are shown in figure 1 for CAVH systems with either 15 or 20 cm length catheters. For systems with 1.0-mm ID catheters, use of 20-cm catheters results in a 21% reduction in bloodflow as compared to that bloodflow when 15-cm catheters are used. This catheter-length-related drop in bloodflow is only 2% for catheters of 3.0 mm ID.

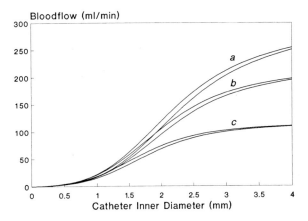

Fig. 1. Predictions of bloodflow through three CAVH systems. Each pair of curves represents bloodflow in a CAVH system with catheter lengths of 20 cm (upper curve) and 15 cm (lower curve). System *a* is a CAVH system with very low end-to-end resistance. System *b* is typical of many CAVH hemofilters available today. System *c* is one of the earlier used CAVH systems with a high end-to-end flow resistance.

Discussion

The effect of variation in catheter length and ID on bloodflow are shown in figure 1 for several commercial CAVH systems. For systems with small diameter catheters (less than 2.0 mm), inner diameter of catheter is the major determinant of bloodflow, with catheter length being of significant but lesser importance. This is expected since resistance varies as the fourth power of diameter, but only as the first power with respect to length of a tube. The hemofilter flow resistance has little effect on system bloodflow, demonstrating the high resistance of these small catheters compared to the remaining system components. Choice of catheter is critical when restricted to small ID catheters. Variability of ID in these catheters is a clinical problem since ID can vary as much as 37% with resultant bloodflow variation as much as 370% [5]. CAVH systems using catheters less than 1.0 mm ID are unlikely to yield adequate bloodflow, even in small infants.

Adult systems will require catheters of at least 2.0 mm ID but 2.5–3.0 mm catheters will yield much higher bloodflows and resultant ultrafiltration rate. For larger diameter catheters, end-to-end hemofilter flow resistance becomes an increasingly more important determinant of system bloodflow. With higher resistance systems, little is gained by increasing the catheter ID over 2.5 mm. The effect of catheter length becomes insignificant with larger catheter ID. Hemofilter resistance, not catheter resistance, becomes the major resistance to flow. We have not dealt with the effect of tip dimension on CAVH bloodflow. We recognize that this effect can be substantial, particularly with catheters not intended for use in CAVH systems.

References

1   Olbricht CH, Schurek H, Stolte H, Koch KM: The influence of vascular access on the efficiency of CAVH; in Sieberth HG, Mann H (eds): Continuous Arteriovenous Hemofiltration. Basel, Karger, 1984, pp 14–24.
2   Kramer P, Gaufhold G, Grone HJ, Wigger W, Rieger J, Matthaei D, Stokke T, Burchardi H, Scheler F: Management of anuric intensive-care patients with arteriovenous hemofiltration. Int J Artif Organs 1980;3:225–230.
3   Lauer A, Saccaggi A, Ronco C, Belledonne M, Glabman S, Bosch JP: Continuous arteriovenous hemofiltration in the critically ill patient. Ann Intern Med 1983;99:455–460.
4   Pallone TL, Petersen JP: Continuous arteriovenous hemofiltration: An in vitro simulation and mathematical model. Kidney Int 1988;33:685–698.
5   Jenkins RD, Kuhn RJ, Funk JE: Clinical implications of catheter variability on neonatal continuous arteriovenous hemofiltration. ASAIO Trans 1988;11:108–111.

Dr. Randall Jenkins, Department of Pediatrics, School of Medicine, University of Louisville, Louisville, KY 40292 (USA)

Sieberth HG, Mann H, Stummvoll HK (eds): Continuous Hemofiltration.
Contrib Nephrol. Basel, Karger, 1991, vol 93, pp 175–178

Importance of Hollow-Fiber Geometry in Continuous Arteriovenous Hemofiltration

*C. Ronco, A. Brendolan, C. Crepaldi, R. Dell'Aquila, M. Milan,
G. La Greca*

Department of Nephrology, St. Bortolo Hospital, Vicenza, Italy

Continuous arteriovenous hemofiltration (CAVH) operates under conditions of low blood flow (Q_b), low transmembrane pressure and high filtration fraction [1]. At a given point inside the filter the oncotic pressure may equal the hydrostatic forces, producing a 'filtration pressure equilibrium' and leading to easy clotting, low efficiency and consequent failure of the CAVH treatment [2]. These problems have been at least partially solved by the introduction of different treatment modalities [3 – 6]. In this study, a new polysulfone fiber has been developed and utilized in two new devices for CAVH with higher ultrafiltration capacities and lower resistance to blood flow (hemofilter D20n and D30n, Amicon, Danvers, Mass., USA). They were compared with the similar units containing the traditional polysulfone fiber (D20 and D30).

Methods

In vitro experiments were carried out on 12 hemofilters (D20n, D20, D30n, D30) in order to test the hydraulic properties, the permeability characteristics, the adequacy of the structure of the filter and the blood path geometry to operate under conditions of arteriovenous pressure gradients as required in CAVH treatment. The following experiments were performed: (1) measurement of blood flows through the device at different inlet hydrostatic pressures, by allowing blood flow into the hemofilter from a reservoir placed at different heights; (2) measurement of the hydrostatic pressures at the inlet and outlet of the blood compartment at different blood flows generated by a pump, to describe the pressure drop inside the fibers; (3) measurement of spontaneous filtration rates achieved at different blood flows, and (4) measurement of ultrafiltration rates (UFRs) at different transmembrane pressures with a blood flow of 250 ml/min to compute ultrafiltration coefficient (K_f) and to calculate the hydraulic permeability of the membrane (K_o).

In vivo studies have been performed on 6 patients with acute renal failure and severe cardiovascular instability using D20n and D30n for CAVH. The operative parameters of the filters have been recorded over 24 h of treatment. In all cases, for few hours, dialysate was circulated in the ultrafiltrate compartment in CAVHD mode to evaluate the diffusive performance of the new fiber.

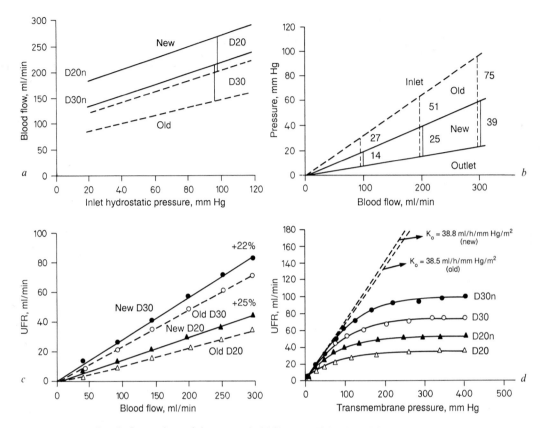

Fig. 1. Comparison of the new and old fibers. *a* Higher blood flows are achieved at the same perfusion pressure (average values: D20n = 48 – 62% increase in Q_b, D30n = 43 – 61% increase in Q_b; venous pressure = 0). *b* The end-to-end pressure drop inside the filter is dramatically reduced (54%; D20 device). *c* Spontaneous filtration at a given blood flow is slightly increased. *d* Membrane K_f (K_o) is almost the same and the final improvement in filtration mostly depends on the larger surface area.

Results

The data given in figure 1 can be explained as follows. The new filters show a lower intrinsic resistance than the previous ones, demonstrated by: (1) high blood flows through the devices at different hydrostatic pressure, and (2) a lower pressure drop inside the hollow fibers. (3) The larger cross-sectional area of the new devices produces a significant reduction of filtration as a function of blood flow, the final effect being only a 22 and 25% increase in the D30n and D20n filters, respectively. (4) The new devices show remarkable filtration rates when transmembrane pressure is

Table 1. CAVH treatment parameters

Patient	Filter	MAP mm Hg	UF pressure neg., mm Hg	Blood flow ml/min	UFR ml/min	Filtration fraction, %
M.A.	D30n	80	40	120	18	22.5
S.B.	D20n	70	40	115	14	15.6
G.A.	D20n	55	45	95	12	17.1
V.P.	D30n	90	50	137	21	21.0
D.M.	D20n	75	40	85	10	16.6
B.D.	D30n	60	45	104	16	24.6

The results are average values of the first 12 h of treatment. MAP = Mean arterial pressure.

progressively increased. The hydraulic permeability of the new membrane and the calculated membrane ultrafiltration coefficient (K_o) remain identical to the previous one, and the higher performances are mostly related to the increased surface area.

Some operational parameters, recorded during the first 12 h of CAVH treatment, are reported in table 1. Despite high UFRs, the higher blood flows achieved permitted the filtration fractions to be adequate to avoid clotting of the filter and even reduce the heparin requirement. Urea clearances up to 30 ml/min were achieved with an average dialysate flow of 40 ml/min.

Discussion

In CAVH, blood flow is a function of the resistance since no pumps are used. The goal of an adequate CAVH device is to achieve the highest blood flow at a given arteriovenous pressure gradient. The new fiber with increased cross-sectional area, reduces the resistance by about 60%. The increase in UFRs observed can be explained by a larger surface area and by a higher blood flow. The increased inner diameter of the fibers does not reduce the wall shear rates and allows for a better performance of filters also in diffusive mode since higher blood flows are permitted. We think that this approach represents one of the first attempts to design specific CAVH-oriented devices.

References

1   Lauer A, Saccaggi A, Ronco C, Belledonne M, Glabman S, Bosch JP: Continuous arteriovenous hemofiltration in the critically ill patient. Ann Intern Med 1986;99:455 – 460.

2   La Greca G, Fabris A, Ronco C: Proc Int Symp on Continuous Arteriovenous Hemofiltration, Vicenza 1986. Milano, Wichtig, 1986.

3   Ronco C, Brendolan A, Bragantini L, Chiaramonte S, Feriani L, Fabris A, La Greca G:
     Continuous arteriovenous haemofiltration; in Berlyne GM, Giovannetti S (eds): Contrib
     Nephrol. Basel, Karger, 1985, vol 48, pp 70–88.
4   Ronco C, Brendolan A, Bragantini L, Fabris A, Feriani M, Chiaramonte S, Fecondini
     L, La Greca G: Studies on blood flow dynamic and ultrafiltration kinetics during
     continuous arteriovenous hemofiltration. Blood Purif 1986;4:220.
5   Olbricht CJ, Schurek HJ, Tytul S, Muller C, Stolte H: Comparison between Scribner
     shunt and femoral catheters as vascular access for continuous arteriovenous hemofiltra-
     tion; in Kramer P (ed): Arteriovenous Hemofiltration. Berlin, Springer, 1985, pp 57–66.
6   Olbricht CJ, Schurek HJ, Stolte H, Koch KM: The influence of vascular access modes
     on the efficiency of CAVH; in Sieberth HG, Mann H (eds): Continuous Arteriovenous
     Hemofiltration. Basel, Karger, 1985, pp 14 – 24.

Dr. Claudio Ronco, Department of Nephrology, St. Bortolo Hospital,
I–36100 Vicenza (Italy)

Sieberth HG, Mann H, Stummvoll HK (eds): Continuous Hemofiltration.
Contrib Nephrol. Basel, Karger, 1991, vol 93, pp 179–183

Ultrafiltration and Pressure Profiles in Continuous Arteriovenous Hemofiltration Studied by Computerized Scintigraphic Imaging

C. Ronco[a], *A. Lupi*[b], *A. Brendolan*[a], *M. Feriani*[a], *G. La Greca*[a]

Departments of [a]Nephrology and [b]Nuclear Medicine, St. Bortolo Hospital, Vicenza, Italy

Continuous arteriovenous hemofiltration (CAVH) is a treatment that operates in conditions of low blood flow and low transmembrane pressure [1]. Clotting of the filters during treatment is mostly correlated with a progressive increase in hematocrit and protein concentration. When inside the filter oncotic pressure equalizes hydrostatic pressure a filtration pressure equilibrium (FPE) occurs, resulting in high resistance to blood flow and frequent clotting of fibers [2]. Depending on blood flow and hydraulic filtration pressure (blood + ultrafiltration pressures), this phenomenon occurs at different degrees of filtration fraction and in different points of the filter. To avoid this, filters with different geometry have been created [3] to adapt the device to the conditions of blood flow.

In this paper, scintigraphic computerized imaging is utilized to demonstrate the occurrence of the FPE phenomenon.

Methods

Six Amicon D30 hemofilters were studied in this protocol utilizing the in vitro circuit depicted in figure 1. Blood with an average hematocrit of 30% was circulated by gravity at different flows (50, 75, 100, 110, 130 and 150 ml/min) through the filter. The arterial and venous reservoirs as well as the ultrafiltrate bag were placed at a fixed height in order to maintain the hydrostatic pressure constant.

Hydrostatic pressures were measured at the blood and ultrafiltrate ports by digital manometers (Digi-dyne, Renal Systems, Minneapolis, Minn., USA). The filters were placed on the horizontal support of the scan and securely fixed to the collimator. Albumin macroaggregates with a molecular diameter ranging from 10 to 90 μm, labeled with metastable 99Tc, were utilized as a nondiffusible marker substance (Macrotec, Sorin Biomedica, Saluggia, Italy). The ultrafiltrate was controlled on-line with a Geiger-Müller counter to evaluate any possible leak of the marker molecule across the membrane. At steady state, the scintigraphic pattern of the dialyzer was acquired utilizing a Toshiba GCA 90b

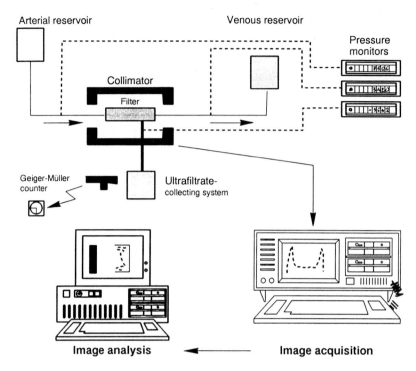

Fig. 1. Circuit utilized for the in vitro experiments. Blood is circulated by gravity from the arterial to the venous reservoir. Radiolabeled albumin is added to the blood and the filter is placed on the collimator of a gamma camera. Once the image has been acquired, it is elaborated on a separate console to obtain the curves of concentration of the marker molecule. To ensure that the molecule has not been filtrated across the membrane the Geiger-Müller counter is continuously scanning the ultrafiltrate-collecting bag.

Gamma camera, equipped with a LEAP collimator. The images obtained in different conditions were elaborated to obtain a detailed profile of the percent changes in concentration of the tracer throughout the length of the filter. Local water fluxes were calculated in each single segment of the dialyzer on the basis of the percent changes in concentration of the tracer.

Cumulative ultrafiltration was measured by timed collection and calculated by the formula:

$$Q_f = Q_{bi}(1 - C_1/C_2),$$

where: Q_f = ultrafiltration rate; Q_b = blood flow (i = inlet); C_1 = lowest count value at the inlet of the dialyzer behind the arterial blood port, and C_2 = highest count value inside the dialyzer. The profile of ultrafiltration throughout the length of the dialyzer $[Q_f = f(l)]$ is defined by the ratio of dQ_f/dl. This ratio is governed by the marker concentration profile

Table 1. Scintigraphic calculation of ultrafiltration (Q_f), pressure (P_{b_i}, P_{b_o} and P_{UF}) and filtration fraction (FF) profiles at different blood flows (Q_b)

Q_b ml/min	Q_f ml/min	P_{b_i} mm Hg	P_{b_o} mm Hg	P_{UF} mm Hg	FF %
50	7.0	20	15	−30	20.0
75	10.4	25	15	−30	19.9
100	13.9	30	15	−30	19.9
110	15.3	33	15	−30	19.8
130	16.5	38	15	−30	18.1
150	18.7	45	15	−30	17.8

defined by the ratio dc/dl. Therefore, the local ultrafiltration can be identified by the ratio dc/dl that represents the variation in concentration of the marker molecule in a single element of dialyzer length. The integration of these ratios for the entire length of the dialyzer permits to derive a curve for the ultrafiltration profile. When the marker molecule concentration is constant no more ultrafiltration takes place. This condition implies a filtration pressure close to zero and FPE.

Results

The 6 filters tested displayed the same behavior in terms of blood flow, pressure drop and ultrafiltration rate at a given perfusion pressure. The experimental data were collected to permit a comparison between the observed ultrafiltration (Q_f) and filtration fraction and the same parameters calculated by the scintigraphic method. Since the values of Q_f and filtration fraction were comparable with the two methods, the calculation of the punctual ultrafiltration and transmembrane pressure made from the scintigraphic image was considered acceptable. Table 1 summarizes these data in detail. In figure 2, three curves relevant to 75, 110 and 150 ml/min of blood flow are shown. The nondiffusible marker molecule (albumin) displays a progressive increase in concentration, reaching a plateau at different points inside the filter, depending on blood flow (fig. 2a). In figure 2b, the behavior of ultrafiltration is shown. At $Q_b = 75$, Q_f stops at 8 cm from the filter inlet, at $Q_b = 110$, Q_f stops at about 12 cm, and at $Q_b = 150$, Q_f tends to zero at the filter outlet. The transmembrane pressure inside the filter is shown in figure 2c. When the hydrostatic and the oncotic pressure become equal, ultrafiltration ceases and FPE is achieved. The curves presented in figure 2 were chosen because FPE is reached inside the fibers at a point corresponding approximately to the length of the D10 and D20 hemofilters (9.5 and 12.7 cm, respectively).

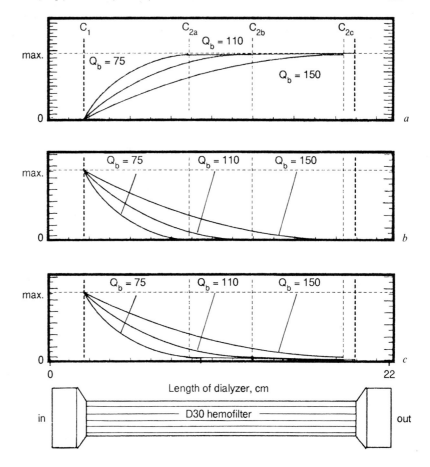

Fig. 2. Profile of radiolabeled albumin concentration *(a)*, and derived profiles of ultrafiltration *(b)* and pressure *(c)* for three different blood flows. The curves reach the plateau corresponding to the FPE point at different distances from the filter inlet. Filtration fraction in these cases was constant.

Discussion

In this study, the occurrence of FPE has been experimentally demonstrated. The new method appears to be reliable to detect the profiles of pressure and ultrafiltration inside hollow-fiber devices. In previous experiments, the constancy of filtration fractions at various blood flows was an indirect proof of FPE but the exact point where this phenomenon occurs inside the filter can only be seen with this new technique. The utility of this method consists in the indication of the minimal blood flow necessary to avoid FPE in a filter of a given length, thus reducing the heparin requirement and the risk of clotting. Finally, this method may be useful for the design of new devices specifically oriented to operate in continuous therapies.

References

1   Lauer A, Saccaggi A, Ronco C, Belledonne M, Glabman S, Bosch JP: Continuous arterio-venous hemofiltration in the critically ill patient. Ann Intern Med 1983;99:455–460.
2   Ronco C, Brendolan A, Bragantini M, Chiaramonte S, Feriani M, Fabris A, La Greca G: Self-limited dehydration during CAVH. Blood Purif 1984;2:88–92.
3   Ronco C, Bosch JP, Lew S, Fecondini L, Brendolan A, Bragantini L, Chiaramonte S, Feriani M, Fabris A, La Greca G: Technical and clinical evaluation of a new hemofilter for CAVH: Theoretical concepts and practical application of a different blood flow geometry; in La Greca G, Fabris A, Ronco C (eds): Proc Int Symp on Continuous Arteriovenous Hemofiltration, Vicenza 1986. Milano, Wichtig, 1986, pp 55–59.

Dr. Claudio Ronco, Department of Nephrology, St. Bortolo Hospital,
I–36100 Vicenza (Italy)

Sieberth HG, Mann H, Stummvoll HK (eds): Continuous Hemofiltration.
Contrib Nephrol. Basel, Karger, 1991, vol 93, pp 184–192

Automated Fluid Balance in Continuous Hemodialysis with Blood Safety Module BSM 22/VPM

K. Sodemann, A. Niedenthal, A. Russ, C. Weber, G.E. Schäfer

Medizinische Klinik III, Städtische Kliniken, Offenbach am Main, FRG

Continuous hemo*filtration* (CHF) is a procedure which requires an accurate control of fluid balance. This work usually is done by the nursing staff in the intensive care unit (ICU). Every hour or sometimes more often the nurse reads (1) the amount of fluid removal in the urinary bag by volumetric control. Then she calculates (2) the achieved fluid balance with regard (3) to the influx of substitution fluid in the last hour and adjusts (4) the infusion pump due to the predetermined filtrate volume of the next hour. Each of these four steps might be a source of error.

As a result, a mechanical device [1] and some microprocessor-controlled gravimetric appliances [2] have been developed in previous years, but they are not widespread partially because of their expensiveness.

In continuous hemo*dialysis* (CHD) a fixed flow of dialysate (Q_d) of usually 1 liter/h simplifies monitoring of balance. There are only two steps: first, measuring the volume of the dialysate outlet (i.e. infused dialysate + a variable amount of filtrate) and second, changing the adjustable height of the collecting bag (deep = more filtrate; high = less filtrate) according to the desired fluid removal. In addition, due to high hydraulic permeability of the hemofilter an excess of filtrate is obtained and enables an automated fluid balance even in spontaneous procedure (arteriovenous hemodialysis, CAVHD).

A well-known and simple principle for *isovolumetric* balance [3] is simultaneous application of *two tubings* of identical inner diameter inserted into *one pump head* realized in former years by Nipro for hemofiltration and Fresenius for plasmapheresis. We applied this technique [4] to CAVHD and continuous venovenous hemodialysis (CVVHD) using double pump blood safety module BSM 22/VPM (Hospal). After extensive laboratory tests concerning adequacy of fluid balance including usual infusion pumps, we made a clinical evaluation in 96 patients from August 88 to August 90.

Study Protocol

(1) In laboratory tests we checked the exactness of various *infusion pumps* being common practice in the ICU for balancing substitution fluid respectively dialysate.

(2) In a *simulation model* the accuracy of the automated fluid balancing system by simultaneous insertion of two tubings to one pump head was tested in a permanent trial over a period of 52 days. The following parts of the system were varied in order to recognize their influence on precision of balance: tubings, pressure in the inlet and outlet of dialysate, flow of dialysate, filters with different ultrafiltration factor, pump heads, and pump module.

(3) The precision of the isovolumetric balance was protocolled in 8 patients in CAVHD and 8 tests in CVVHD changing the ultrafiltration from 0 ml/h up to 300 ml/h.

(4) In 96 patients (41 CAVHD, 55 CVVHD) on 667 days of treatment automated fluid balance was applied on the ICU *without any alternative control*. Hourly fluid removal by ultrafiltration was determined in stages of 50 ml/h up to 500 ml/h under clinical aspects by the medical staff.

Methods and Material

Infusion Pump

The tested infusion pumps were in routine use of ICU since 2 years. One model was Volumed (Fresenius, 4 appliances) with an infusion rate from 1 to 999 ml/h, the other device Intramat 1000 (MSB, 2 appliances) with an infusion rate from 1 to 5,000 ml/h. For every test new tubes were applied (Intradrop Air VS or Intradrop Air P; Fresenius). Substitution fluid (SH 21, Schiwa) in a 4,500-ml bag was infused with an infusion rate of 999 or 1,000 ml/h. The fluid was collected in another bag hung up 70 cm below the infusion pump (fig. 1). The exactness of pumps was controlled continuously by two electronical sales (Infusart; Sartorius). Time related changes of infusion rate were protocolled comparing the infused volume indicated on the display of the infusion pump and the really pumped amount controlled by the scales. Differences were calculated in percentages. The trial was broken off after infusion of the bag (4,500 ml).

Laboratory Tests of BSM 22/VPM

The automated fluid balancing system was achieved by inserting two tubings with a 4-mm inner diameter of pump segment to 'balance input/output' (BIO) pump of BSM 22 (Hospal); this allows an isovolumetric control of dialysate flow (Q_d) by a closed system. The pump head of BIO pump was modified by stronger springs in order to improve occlusion up to 400 mm Hg. Pressures in all sections of dialysate tubings were controlled and adjusted to 70 mm Hg by clamps. For monitoring isovolumetric balance the dialysate recirculated in a half-filled bag controlled by electronical scales (Infusart). In the laboratory test we simulated blood flow by recirculation of sodium chloride solution 0.9% in blood compartment of the filter with a flow of 70 ml/min; a pressure of 70 mm Hg in venous pressure chamber was achieved by a clamp (fig. 2). A shift of fluid from blood to dialysate compartment or vice versa was checked in a long-term trial each time over a period of 24 h gravimetrically controlled by the two scales. Differences were calculated in percentages with regard to the absolute amount of pumped dialysate (Q_d was 1,000 or 2,000 ml/h). In the immediately following test only one factor was modified in order to notice influences possibly affecting adequacy of balance, such as variations of inner diameter of tubings or pressure differences in the inlet and outlet of dialysate. To compensate the effect of a decreased pressure in the dialysate conveying tube the pressure was increased by a clamp in the drain line. Four highly permeable filters were tested with different ultrafiltration factor and surface (AV 400, AV 600/Fresenius and Multiflow 60, Filtral 10/Hospal).

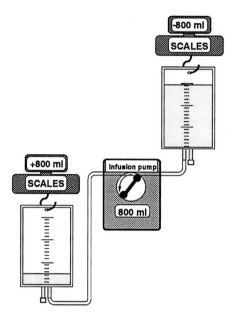

Fig. 1. Gravimetric control of exactness of infusion pumps.

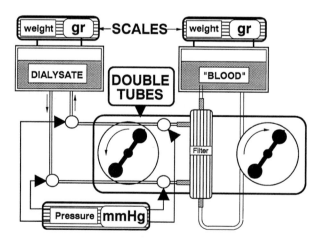

Fig. 2. Gravimetric control of automated fluid balance in simulation model.

Clinical Tests of BSM 22/VPM

(1) *CAVHD:* In CAVHD, BSM 22 exclusively controls dialysate flow and fluid removal; the blood pump is not required (fig. 3a). Therefore the two tubings for isovolumetric balance are inserted to the head of the blood pump (modified by stronger springs). This pump is calibrated to a pump segment of 8 mm inner diameter indicating in the display a value which has to be divided by 4 to get the real flow in ml/min. An indicated flow of 70 ml/min results in 17.5 ml/min corresponding to a dialysate flow of 1,050 ml/h. Elevating Q_d improves detoxification. The usual adjustment was 70 ml/min (1 liter/h), as an exception Q_d was increased up to 150 ml/min, i.e. approximately 2 liters/h. Fluid level of dialysate in the bags is controlled by venous pressure monitor (VPM) triggering a stop of the pump and an audible alarm in empty bags. Volume depletion is managed by fitting a Y-connection into dialysate outlet of the filter connected to a 4-mm tubing inserted in the BIO pump. Fluid removal can be controlled in stages of 50 ml/h from 0 up to 2,000 ml/h. The current adjustment is indicated permanently. The pressure monitor of the BIO pump was focused by a technician on -150 to $+150$ mm Hg (usually from 0 to 300 mm Hg), so that a sucking of filtrate is possible up to a negative pressure of 150 mm Hg. If the filter is clotting, the BIO pump triggers an alarm due to the adjusted alarm limits. Transmembranous pressure (TMP) is indicated permanently in the display.

Isovolumetric balance of dialysate was controlled in the same manner as in the infusion pumps. Q_d was varied from 1 to 2 liters/h. Checked by two scales, differences of dialysate inlet and outlet were protocolled under different rates of ultrafiltration (0, 50, 100 and 200 ml/h), divergences were calculated in percentages. All patients were treated with the filter Multiflow 60 (membrane AN 69 HF, surface 0.6 m², Hospal).

(2) *CVVHD:* In CVVHD, BSM 22 controls blood flow (Q_b) commonly in the range of 60–100 ml/min. Isovolumetric balance is achieved by BIO pump as described above (fig. 3b). For fluid removal, dialysate outlet is connected by a Y-connection with an additional infusion pump (Intramat, MSB). TMP is registered by VPM with a second Y-connection in dialysate inlet of filter. Q_b is adjusted according to the fluid removal, so that a positive TMP always exists. A filtrate sucking by the infusion pump is unnecessary under these conditions.

Pressure in dialysate outlet has to be adjusted by a tubing because of the positive TMP. A hydrophobic filter in the top of the adjustable tube interrupts the pillar of fluid and lets dialysate drop into the tank under the BSM 22. Accuracy of balance was tested under the same conditions as in CAVHD with two electronical scales in dialysate inlet and outlet by varying Q_d and ultrafiltration.

Clinical Evaluation

From August 1988 to August 1990, all patients of the two ICUs of our hospital with acute renal failure complicated by cardiovascular instability were treated by CHD using automated fluid balance with BSM 22/VPM. The decision on arteriovenous or venovenous procedure was made usually for organization reasons. With the exception of overhydrated patients, hourly fluid removal was commonly fixed at 150 ml/h due to generous parenteral nutrition. Some patients with nonoliguric renal failure were treated without volume depletion.

Results

Infusion Pumps

Infusing 4,500 ml of dialysate 6 times by every tested infusion pump showed the following results (fig 4a). Flow rate error had a range of $-5.9 \pm 1.43\%$ to $+3.8 \pm 0.93\%$. Four of the 6 pumps had an error near

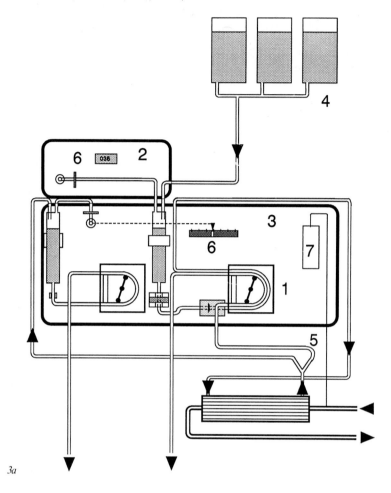

3a

2% or lower. At beginning of infusion error was larger and remained stable
after 2 h.

Simulation Test of CVVHD without Ultrafiltration

The mean deviation from isovolumetric balance was in the range of
$-0.6 \pm 0.28\%$ to $-1.3 \pm 0.78\%$ (fig 4b). One trial lasted 24 h on average
and was carried out 8 times under identical conditions. The total time of
the test period was 52 days. Changing the PVC tubings showed no
influence on the balance. If the pressures in dialysate inlet and outlet were
the same, no difference was recognized. Elevating pressure in the draining

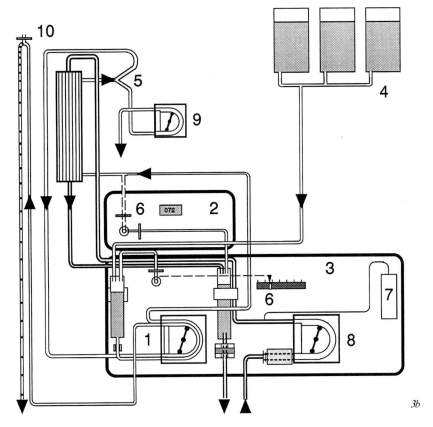

Fig. 3. Flow diagrams of *a* CAVHD and *b* CVVHD: 1 = double tubings in pump head; 2 = VPM; 3 = BSM 22; 4 = dialysate; 5 = Y-connection; 6 = pressure control; 7 = heparin pump; 8 = blood pump; 9 = infusion pump; 10 = hydrophobic filter.

line from 70 to 100 mm Hg was compensated by lowering the pressure in the conveying tube by the same amount. Under these conditions the deviation was $-1.1 \pm 0.66\%$ resp. $-1.3 \pm 0.78\%$ on average by a Q_d of 1.0 resp. 2.0 liters/h.

Balance Control under Clinical Conditions

(1) *CAVHD:* The mean divergence of isovolumetric balance varied from $1.4 \pm 0.82\%$ to $2.8 \pm 1.16\%$ (fig. 5a). Every stage of ultrafiltration was controlled in 8 patients over a period of 30 min. The results are shown in the diagrams due to the different dialysate flow (fig. 5b).

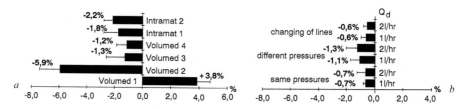

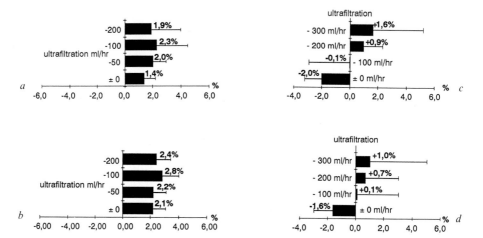

Fig. 4. a Flow error of different infusion pumps. *b* Deviation of isovolumetric balance varying pressures, lines, and Q_d in BSM 22/VPM.

Fig. 5. Divergence of isovolumetric balance (n = 8) in *a* CAVHD, Q_d = 1.0 liter/h; *b* CAVHD, Q_d = 2.0 liter/h; *c* CVVHD, Q_d = 1.0 liter/h; *d* CVVHD, Q_d = 2.0 liter/h.

(2) *CVVHD:* In CVVHD, control of balance had a range from $-2.0 \pm 1.18\%$ in zero ultrafiltration to $+1.6 \pm 3.57\%$ in a fluid removal of 300 ml/h (fig. 5c). Controls were made in 8 patients varying the dialysate flow (fig. 5d).

Clinical Evaluation of Automated Fluid Balance

From August 1988 to August 1990, 96 patients were treated with balanced CHD applying BSM 22/VPM on 667 days. Mean duration of treatment was 7 days, min. 1 day, max. 42 days. Survival rate was 32% (31 patients) due to multiple organ failure. Forty-one patients were treated by CAVHD on 437 days (on average 10.7 days) and 55 patients on 230 days (mean 4.2 days) by CVVHD. Fluid removal fitted the clinical requirements. In fluid overload the amount of depleted volume was up to 10 liters/day. Some patients with nonoliguric renal failure were treated by zero ultrafiltration using sterile dialysate in countercurrent flow. In CAVHD, alarms very seldom occurred. In CVVHD, because of pump-assisted blood circulation, there were about 8 alarms/day, especially while bedding the patient.

Discussion
Infusion Pumps

The laboratory tests show a wide variation in the accuracy of the pumps. One pump for example has a difference of 3.8% on average which results in a positive fluid balance of 40 ml/h in contrast to what is indicated on the display. In this manner the patient has an unnoticed fluid load of 1,000 ml/day. Another pump has a deviation of 5.3% on average with an unobserved negative balance of approximately 1,250 ml/day. Nearly all pumps transported less fluid than displayed in spite of sucking by the drawing-off tube (70 cm H_2O) and positive pressure of the infusion bag (70 cm H_2O at beginning of infusion). Each of the pumps seems to be stable in its error in the laboratory test. The deviation of the two roller pumps (Intramat) is lower, usually near 2%. If an infusion pump is used in CHD, the properties of the appliance should be known for example by previous volumetric control. A permanent gravimetric surveillance by two scales would be preferable.

Laboratory Tests of BSM 22/VPM

Adjusting pressures in the tubings the precision of fluid control was adequate. Due to high quality of the PVC lines we did not observe any variations of fluid balance. Dialysate flow can be increased up to 2 liters/h without any influence.

Clinical Tests

In CAVHD may result a positive fluid balance up to 2%, that means 20 ml/h in a dialysate flow of 1,000 ml/h. This imbalance can be simply compensated by increasing the fluid removal by the BIO pump. At any rate, the range was lower than the doctor's ability in estimating the patient's correct hydration status. Among the staff we had more discussions whether fluid removal should be 50 or 150 ml/h than any skepticism about the accuracy of balance.

In CVVHD an adjustment of pressure can be achieved by a pillar of fluid in the draining tube. Under these conditions the divergence is less than 1% in ultrafiltration rate between 100 and 200 ml/h. The balancing pump has to be modified by stronger springs because of the positive pressure in the dialysate circuit.

Clinical Evaluation

Balanced CHD was applied in nearly 100 patients in more than 600 days of treatment. No detrimental imbalance occurred in long-term modalities though automated fluid balance was applied without any further volumetric or gravimetric control. The system seems to be safer than the conventional method of measuring and calculating by the nursing staff. It has a good acceptance by simplifying their work.

Conclusion

Using BSM 22/VPM an automated fluid-balancing system can be established in CHD even in spontaneous procedure (CAVHD). It can be applied in long-term renal replacement therapy in the ICU and it is satisfactory to clinical requirements. It is safe, reliable and needs little surveillance.

References

1   Schurek HJ, Biela JD, Bergmann KH: Further improvement of a mechanical device for automatic fluid balance in CAVH; in Sieberth HG, Mann H (eds): Continuous Arteriovenous Hemofiltration (CAVH). Int. Conf on CAVH, Aachen 1984. Basel, Karger, 1985, pp 67–75.
2   Schultheis R, Brings W, Glöckner WM, Sieberth H-G: Device for controlled cyclic substitution during spontaneous filtration; in Sieberth HG, Mann H (eds): Continuous Arteriovenous Hemofiltration (CAVH). Int Conf on CAVH, Aachen 1984. Basel, Karger, 1985, pp 64–66.
3   Yamagami S, Yoshimoto S, Ota M, Tanaka H, Kishimoto T, Maekawa M, Sano M: An automatic controlled hemofiltration system and the clinical evaluation. Artif Organs (Japan) 1978;7:279.
4   Sodemann K, Schäfer GE, Schröder H-M, Eckrich W, Schuh N, Förster H: Vorteile der bilanzierten kontinuierlichen arterio- bzw. veno-venösen Hämodialyse (CAVHD/CVVHD). Klin Wochenschr 1989;67(suppl 16):133–134.

Dr. K. Sodemann, Medizinische Klinik III, Städtische Kliniken,
Starkenburgring 66, D–W–6050 Offenbach am Main (FRG)

Sieberth HG, Mann H, Stummvoll HK (eds): Continuous Hemofiltration.
Contrib Nephrol. Basel, Karger, 1991, vol 93, pp 193–195

Microfilter for Drawing Plasma Samples from the Extracorporeal Circulation

S. Stiller [a], *H. Mann* [b]

Medical Clinic [a]III and [b]II, Technical University, Aachen, FRG

Clinical laboratory investigations concerning dialysis therapy often require repeated measurements of plasma concentrations of substances like electrolytes, uremic toxins, hormones, enzymes, etc. However, taking blood samples frequently from anemic patients increases renal anemia and is often refused by the patients. This problem can be avoided when taking plasma samples through a microfilter instead of whole blood. For such applications small and cheap (< $20) plasma filters have been developed and are described here in detail.

Construction of the Filter

Two types of filter are available: the filter is either an independent module which can subsequently be integrated anywhere in the extracorporeal circuit or it is integrated within the tubing system by the manufacturer (manufactured and sold by Meise Medizintechnik, Gewerbering 15, D–5885 Schalksmühle, FRG). The standard model contains 11 filter capillaries (Enka Plasmaphan P1 LX; inner diameter 330 μm, wall thickness 150 μm, length 35 cm, maximum pore size 0.4–0.6 μm), which are closed at one end. The closed end drifts freely in the bloodstream of the extracorporeal blood circuit. The open end of the capillaries is connected to a Luer connector for drawing filtrate (fig. 1). As there are only 11 single capillaries, the filtrate volume (dead space) of this filter is very low (0.05 ml) and the few capillaries only slightly increase flow resistance in the blood tubing.

Using the Filter

Generally the filter will be inserted directly in the arterial line in order to determine the concentrations of blood constituents in the blood coming from the patient. If the clearance of a dialyzer has to be measured in vivo a second microfilter downstream to the dialyzer also can be inserted. The performance of the microfilters is characterized by the filtration rate as a

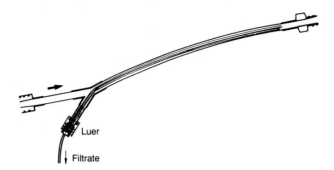

Fig. 1. Micro plasma filter integrated in the blood tubing system or as a separated module. Filtration occurs from outside into the capillary (Enka Plasmaphan P1 LX).

function of transmembrane pressure. The filtrate is normally drawn by a small roller pump. In this case the transmembrane pressure is established according to the filtration rate. The transmembrane pressure needed to obtain a certain filtration rate increases with dialysis time. This is probably the consequence of protein adsorption on the (outer) membrane surface of the capillaries which leads to reduction in pore size. For the same reason, hemolysis starts at a filtration rate of 1.5 ml/min at the start of dialysis and at a rate of 1.8 ml/min after 5 h. Hemolysis also occurs when the blood is flowing inside the capillaries as in normal use for plasma-pheresis. In vitro experiments with bovine blood [1] have shown that hemoglobin concentration and shear rate at the capillary wall are the main influencing parameters. For hematocrit values greater than 34% hemolysis in the microfilters may occur at a filtration rate below 1.5 ml/min, but within common hematocrit ranges of dialysis patients a filtration rate > 1.0 ml/min is easily obtained. The pressure drop in the blood line over the length of the microfilter increases linearly with blood flow rate and reaches a value of 26 mm Hg at a flow rate of 400 ml/min. This means that the filter can always be inserted in the blood stream, even at such high blood flow rates.

Discussion

The determination of blood concentrations is mostly done in plasma or serum. The separation of plasma from erythrocytes by a centrifuge is not necessary if the plasma is drawn directly by filtration. Only a very small amount of plasma, filling the tubing from the filter to the sampling vessel (dead space < 0.1 ml), has to be discarded. Using these filters only the quantity needed for the measurement has to be taken. Therefore, time, erythrocytes, and plasma are saved. Since time for separation is saved, plasma probes can be deep frozen immediately to avoid decay of unstable plasma constituents. This easy-to-use and cheap microsampling filter may offer many possible investigations for further advancing and optimizing dialysis therapy.

Reference

1   Dinc LH, Jaffren MY, Gupta BB: A model of hemolysis in membrane plasmapheresis. Trans Am Soc Artif Intern Organs 1986;32:330–333.

Siegfried Stiller, Dipl.-Physiker, Medical Clinic III, Pauwelsstrasse 30, D–W–5100 Aachen (FRG)

Sieberth HG, Mann H, Stummvoll HK (eds): Continuous Hemofiltration.
Contrib Nephrol. Basel, Karger, 1991, vol 93, pp 196–198

Continuous Arteriovenous Hemodiafiltration: Filter Design and Blood Flow Rate

H.H. Vincent[a], *E. Akcahuseyin*[b], *M.C. Vos*[a], *W.A. van Duyl*[b],
M.A.D.H. Schalekamp[a]

Departments of [a]Internal Medicine and [b]Biomedical Physics and Technology,
Erasmus University, Rotterdam, The Netherlands

Continuous arteriovenous hemodiafiltration (CAVHD) is the most effective form of renal replacement therapy in intensive care patients. Some centers, however, report a high incidence of technical failures, usually due to inadequate blood flow. According to recent literature [1], the blood flow rate that will be obtained may be calculated from filter geometry by applying Poiseuille's law and using a formula for the estimation of blood viscosity. This was borne out by two laboratory studies [1, 2] in which blood flow rate through the hemofilter was within 20% of the predicted value. In clinical studies, however, we and others, using the same methods, have found that blood flow rate was only one-third of the predicted value. Similar discrepancies were found for several different hemofilters, namely, Hospal SCU/CAVH and Multiflow-60, Sorin Spiraflo HFTO2 [3], Amicon D20 and D30, Gambro FH66, Fresenius AV400 [4]. In order to elucidate the possible causes for this discrepancy, we made a detailed study of the 0.6 m² AN-69 capillary filter (Multiflow-60, Hospal, France).

Methods

Patients were treated with CAVHD for acute renal failure and sepsis and/or circulatory, respiratory or neurological instability. For vascular access we used special 8F CAVH catheters (Medcomp) or Scribner shunts (Quinton).

Pre- and postfilter blood pressure, P_{pre} and P_{post}, and the blood flow rate through the filter, Qb, were measured. After clamping the blood line, we also measured intra-arterial pressure, P_{art}. The resistance to blood flow of the arterial access was calculated as $(P_{art}-P_{pre})/$ Qb and the resistance of the hemofilter, Rf, was calculated as $(P_{pre}-P_{post})/Qb$. Hematocrit, Ht, and serum protein concentration, Cp, were determined to estimate blood viscosity, μ, as described by Pallone et al. [2]. We then calculated the normalized filter resistance, Rfn, as Rf/μ. Rfn was also predicted according to Poiseuille's law: $Rfn_{pred} = 8 \cdot L/(N \cdot \pi \cdot r^4)$, where L is the fiber length, N is the number of fibers, and r is the internal fiber radius. In a separate study we took blood from 10 intensive-care patients and measured whole blood viscosity at 37 °C at shear rates similar to those that occur in the filter. Actual viscosity was then compared with the value predicted by the formula.

In the laboratory the hemofilter was perfused with saline, with a viscous sucrose solution and with blood at a range of flow rates. Rf and Rfn were determined.

Results

The average resistance of the CAVH catheter was 10 and that of the hemofilter was 24 (SD 11) mm Hg/100 ml/min. This resulted in an average blood flow rate of 191 (range 107–284) ml/min and an average filter 'survival' of 3 days. The resistance of the Scribner shunt was 36 mm Hg/ 100 ml/min, both at the arterial and at the venous site.

When perfused with blood, the normalized hemofilter resistance to flow, Rfn, was 2.8 and 2.6 times the predicted value under clinical conditions and in the laboratory, respectively. With saline or sucrose, Rfn was only 1.4 times the predicted value.

Actual blood viscosity ranged from 2.27 to 3.17 mPa $\cdot$ s. This was 1.4 (range 1.2–1.5) times higher than according to formula prediction.

Discussion

When using CAVH catheters, filter resistance to blood flow was low enough to obtain an adequate blood flow rate in virtually all patients.

The discrepancy between the predicted and the actual filter resistance was partly due to underestimation of blood viscosity. It would be worthwhile to obtain a greater number of measurements of Ht, Cp and blood viscosity in intensive-care patients in order to develop a better way to estimate blood viscosity. Part of the discrepancy was due to the increased Poiseuille resistance of the filter (measurements with saline and sucrose). This 40% increase of the resistance would be explained by an 8% decrease of the fiber diameter, which is within the accepted range of accuracy. Furthermore, small pressure losses at the hemofilter inlet and outlet might add to the overall filter resistance.

If we would have used actual blood viscosity values and our own laboratory data on the filter resistance, we would have underestimated blood flow rate by no more than 25%. Therefore, we conclude that with a more realistic estimation of blood viscosity and when laboratory data on the Poiseuille resistance are available, a reasonably accurate prediction of blood flow rate through the hemofilter is feasible. This kind of study is helpful in choosing an appropriate type of hemofilter for CAVH or CAVHD.

References

1   Pallone TL, Petersen J: Continuous arteriovenous hemofiltration: An in vitro simulation
    and mathematical model. Kidney Int 1988;33:685–698.
2   Pallone TL, Hyver S, Petersen J: The simulation of continuous arteriovenous hemodial-
    ysis with a mathematical model. Kidney Int 1989;35:125–133.
3   Vincent HH, Akcahuseyin E, Vos MC, van Ittersum FJ, van Duyl WA, Schalekamp
    MADH: Determinants of blood flow and ultrafiltration in continuous arterio-venous
    haemodiafiltration: Theoretical predictions and laboratory and clinical observations.
    Nephrol Dial Transplant 1990;5:1031–1037.
4   Olbricht CJ, Haubitz M, Haebel U, Frei U, Koch K-M: Continuous arteriovenous
    hemofiltration: In vivo functional characteristics and its dependence on vascular accesss
    and filter design. Nephron 1990;55:49–57.

Dr. H.H. Vincent, University Hospital Dijkzigt, Room Bd 338, Dr Molewaterplein 40,
NL–3015 GD Rotterdam (The Netherlands)

Sieberth HG, Mann H, Stummvoll HK (eds): Continuous Hemofiltration.
Contrib Nephrol. Basel, Karger, 1991, vol 93, pp 199–201

Solute Transport in Hemodiafiltration:
A New Mathematical Model to Analyse
Dialyser Performance

H.H. Vincent, M.C. Vos, W.A. van Duyl

Departments of Internal Medicine I and Biomedical Physics and Technology,
Erasmus University, Rotterdam, The Netherlands

Diffusive Mass Transfer Rate (Kd)

When we first developed CAVHD, we were faced with the question
what dialysate flow rate was required to ensure an adequate rate of solute
diffusion. We also wanted to examine the possible impact of protein
adsorption on the rate of diffusion, i.e. we wanted to determine the Kd,
and see if Kd changed in time. To this end, we developed a new mathematical model of hemodiafiltration, based on the equations (see appendix):

$$d(Qwx \cdot Cwx)/dx = -d(Qdx \cdot Cdx)/dx = A/L \cdot Jf \cdot Cwx - A/L \cdot Kd(Cwx - Cdx),$$

which were integrated along the length of the dialyzer. To simplify the
analysis, it was assumed that filtration flux was constant along the length
of the dialyzer. The equations were analytically solved so as to yield an
expression of Kd as a function of membrane surface area and blood,
filtrate and dialysate flow rates and solute concentrations [1].

Effect of Dialysate and Blood Flow Rates on Effective Kd

With our new model we analyzed urea transport in CAVHD. With the
AN-69 0.43 m² plate filter, Pallone et al. [2], in their laboratory study, had
estimated the Kd to be approximately 140 μm/min [2]. With filters that had
been used for less than 12 h, we calculated Kd values between 80 and
200 μm/min. At Qd of 0.5–3.0 liters/h, Kd proved to increase with Qd.
Similar observations were made for other solutes and for other types of
hemofilter. The phenomenon is interpreted to reflect a more homogeneous
distribution of dialysate at higher flow rates, leading to an increase of the
membrane surface area that is effectively available for diffusion.

With the same filter, when blood flow was varied between 50 and
150–200 ml/min while dialysate flow rate was fixed at 3 liters/h, there was

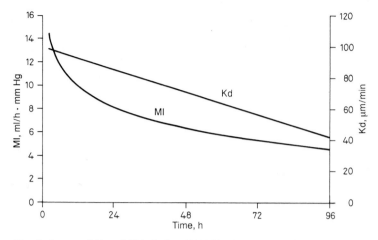

Fig. 1. Average MI and Kd during CAVHD. Data were obtained with the AN-69 0.6 m² capillary dialyzer at a dialysate flow rate of 1 liter/h.

no change in the effective Kd. This contrasts with our findings with other filters in machine hemodialysis, where, at blood flow rates of 50 to 200 ml/min and a dialysate flow rate of 500 ml/min, Kd did increase with Qb. These contrasting findings have so far not been fully explained.

Decrease of Convection and Diffusion in Time

In a study of solute transport by CAVHD [1], we found that the variability of Kd of urea was related not only to differences in Qd but also to the MI. As shown in figure 1, both MI and Kd decrease in time, probably due to ongoing protein adsorption to the membrane.

Relationship between Kd and Molecular Weight

From our studies in CAVHD and from laboratory studies of dialyzer clearance, we calculated Kd values for urea, creatinine, phosphate and vitamin B_{12}. Absolute Kd values varied between studies. Within studies we found a fixed relationship of Kd_{urea}: Kd_{creat}: $Kd_{phosphate}$: $Kd_{B12} = 1.00:0.77:0.62:0.22$. Thus, there was a log-linear correlation between Kd and the solute molecular weight. This relationship was in accordance with theoretical predictions based on Renkin's equation. This relationship may be used for the prediction of drug clearance, either during CAVHD [3] or during intermittent hemodialysis and hemodiafiltration.

Conclusion

Presently, dialyzers are tested by measuring solute clearance rates at a standardized blood and dialysate flow rate. It would, however, be preferable to perform measurements at a range of flow rates. Furthermore, we feel that Kd values are more meaningful than just clearance rates. Kd values may be used to extrapolate findings to different conditions.

Appendix: Definition of Symbols and Units

Q_w = Plasma water flow rate, ml/min; Q_d = dialysate flow rate, ml/min; C_w = solute concentration in plasma water, mmol/l; C_d = solute concentration in dialysate, mmol/l; x = axial coordinate along the fiber, m; L = fiber length, m; A = membrane surface area, m²; J_f = volume flux, μm/min; K_d = diffusive transfer rate, μm/min; M_I = membrane index of ultrafiltration, ml/h· mm Hg.

References

1   Vincent HH, van Ittersum FJ, Akcahuseyin E, Vos MC, van Duyl WA, Schalekamp MADH: Solute transport in continuous arterio-venous hemodiafiltration. A new mathematical model applied to clinical data. Blood Purif 1990;8:149–159.

2   Pallone TL, Hyver S, Petersen J: The simulation of continuous arteriovenous hemodialysis with a mathematical model. Kidney Int 1989;35:125–133.

3   Vos MC, Vincent HH: Continuous arteriovenous hemodiafiltration: Predicting the clearance of drugs; in Sieberth HG, Mann H, Stummvoll HK (eds): Continuous Hemofiltration. Contrib Nephrol. Basel, Karger, 1991, vol 93, pp 143–145.

Dr. H.H. Vincent, Erasmus University Rotterdam, University Hospital Dijkzigt, Room Bd 338, Dr Molewaterplein 40, NL–3015 GD Rotterdam (The Netherlands)

Anticoagulation

Sieberth HG, Mann H, Stummvoll HK (eds): Continuous Hemofiltration.
Contrib Nephrol. Basel, Karger, 1991, vol 93, pp 202–204

Assessment of Standardized Ultrafiltrate Production Rate Using Prostacyclin in Continuous Venovenous Hemofiltration

D. Journois, D. Chanu, P. Pouard, P. Mauriat, D. Safran

Réanimation chirurgicale, Hôpital Laënnec, Paris, France

Continuous hemofiltration (CHF) is a safe and efficient method, widely used as renal replacement therapy in intensive care units. It requires an efficient and continuous anticoagulation to prevent fibrin deposition and thrombus formation leading to early hemofilter clotting. Heparinization could increase the hemorrhagic risk in the postoperative period and in patients with coagulopathies. Topical prostacyclin (PGI_2) infused in the arterial port of the hemofilter as inhibitor of platelet aggregation avoids the use of large doses of heparin, even if low doses are already necessary [1]. The aim of this work was to compare the efficiency of the association of PGI_2 with a low molecular weight heparin (LMWH) versus nonfractionated heparin used alone.

Material and Method

Continuous venovenous hemofiltration used a flat hemofilter (AN-69S Hospal®). Eleven patients with acute renal failure, representing 42 CHF periods, have been randomly included in 2 groups. They received either heparin (9 ± 1 IU/kg · h) (HEP group) or the association of enoxaparin ($25 \pm 4\,\mu g/kg · h$) with PGI_2 (4 ± 0.8 ng/kg · min) (PGI_2 group). Antithrombotic efficiency was appreciated by a hemofilter permeability index (HPI) taking into consideration transmembranous pressure gradient and ultrafiltrate production rate [2]. Hydrostatic (P) and oncotic (Π) pressures were measured over time at the entrance (i), the outlet (o), and in the ultrafiltrate (UF) compartment of the hemofilter. The transmembrane pressure, generating the UF, was calculated as $TMP = 1/2(P_i + P_o) - P_{ur} - 1/2(\Pi_i + \Pi_o)$. UF output was used to define HPI as $HPI = UF/TPM$. Time for HPI to decrease to a third of its initial value ($HPI_{1/3}$) was used to compare these two treatments [3]. Hemodynamics, coagulation profiles (including activated clotting time (ACT), platelet count (PC), bleeding time (BT)), and HPI values were obtained over time.

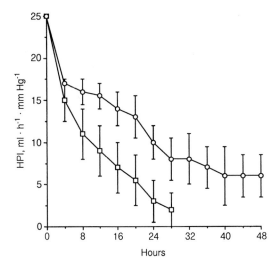

Fig. 1. Evolution over time of the hemofilter permeability index in the heparin (□) and PGI$_2$ + enoxaparin (○) groups.

Results

No adverse effects as bleeding, thrombosis, or hypotension were observed. PGI$_2$ + ENX did not aggravate hemorrhage and no significant changes were observed in hemodynamics. Time to obtain a third of the initial HPI value was 13 ± 3.5 h in the HEP group and 29 ± 3.3 h in the PGI$_2$ group (p < 0.03) (fig. 1). ACT was longer in the HEP group while PC decreased. There was no change in these variables in the PGI$_2$ group at the onset of CHF.

Discussion

PGI$_2$ with LMWH has improved duration of the hemofilter for 55%. In addition, it preserved PC and coagulation profile. Despite PGI$_2$ vasodilator effects, the correct cardiovascular tolerance observed could be explained by PGI$_2$ losses in UF, its short half-life and by the low doses employed. PGI$_2$ could be a good alternative to heparin in a number of patients, above all in those at high risk of hemorrhage. Optimal biological monitoring of these protocols needs further investigations to be determined. The high cost of PGI$_2$ has to be in balance with the increase in hemofiltration duration.

References

1   Zusman RM, Rubin RH, Cato AE, Cocheto DM, Tolkow-Rubin N: Hemodialysis using prostacyclin instead of heparin as the sole antithrombotic agent. N Engl J Med 1981;304:934–939.

2   Pallone TL, Petersen J: Continuous arteriovenous hemofiltration: an in vitro simulation and mathematical model. Kidney Int 1988;33:685–698.

3   Journois D, Safran D, Castelain MH, Chanu D, Drévillon C, Barrier G: Comparaison des effets antithrombotiques de l'héparine, de l'énoxaparine et de la prostacycline au cours de l'hémofiltration continue. Ann Fr Anesth Réanim 1990;9:331–337.

Dr. D. Journois, Réanimation chirurgicale, Hôpital Laënnec,
42, rue de Sèvres, F–75007 Paris (France)

Sieberth HG, Mann H, Stummvoll HK (eds): Continuous Hemofiltration.
Contrib Nephrol. Basel, Karger, 1991, vol 93, pp 205–209

Antithrombotic Management with a Stable Prostacyclin Analogue during Extracorporeal Circulation

Norbert Maurin

Medical Clinic II, University Hospital Aachen, FRG

In certain situations heparin used during extracorporeal circulation can increase the risk of bleeding. Various groups have suggested that this bleeding risk can be reduced by using prostacyclin (PGI_2) [1]. Since PGI_2 is labile under physiological conditions and is thus difficult to use, we have used the stable PGI_2 analogue taprostene (Grünenthal GmbH, Aachen, FRG), which has approximately 20% of the platelet aggregation inhibiting effect of PGI_2 [2] and which is easy to infuse in physiological saline solution. We used hemodialysis (HD) as an example for extracorporeal circulation. The main question for the present study is whether it is possible during 5 h of HD with taprostene to use no heparin at all or at least to markedly reduce the heparin dose.

Methods

This study in 5 chronic HD patients was designed to apply 5 different HD regimens (table 1) with bicarbonate to each patient for 5 h (Cuprophan® capillary dialyzer, double-needle technique, dialysate flow rate 500 ml/min, blood flow rate 150–200 ml/min). Blood count and numerous hemostasis parameters were measured before, during and after HD. In citrated platelet-rich plasma, platelet aggregation after stimulation by ADP (1×10^{-6} mol/l) was determined through the maximum amplitude in the aggregometer test of Born. ECG, blood pressure and pulse were continuously monitored. Any side effects were recorded.

Results

Slight falls in platelets and in some cases substantial falls in leukocytes shortly after commencing HD cannot be avoided when administering taprostene alone.

Both 25 and 35 ng/kg/min doses of taprostene produced approximately 50% inhibition of the ADP-induced platelet aggregation for the entire 5-hour administration period (fig. 1); at 30 min after HD the inhibition had fallen to approximately 20%.

Table 1. Study design

Dialysis No.	Initial bolus dose of heparin IU	Infusion during dialysis	Symbol
1	2,500	heparin (1,875 IU/h)	○
2	—	taprostene (25 ng/kg/min) for the first 120 min, then full heparinization	●
3	—	taprostene (25 ng/kg/min)	□
4	500	heparin (200 IU/h) plus taprostene (25 ng/kg/min)	■
5	500	heparin (200 IU/h) plus taprostene (35 ng/kg/min)	△

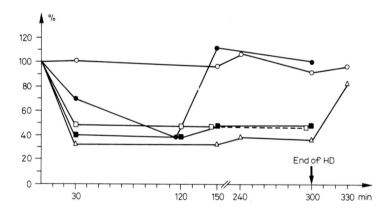

Fig. 1. Inhibition of ADP-induced platelet aggregation (percent of initial level) during dialysis. For explanation of symbols, see table 1.

Although administering taprostene alone for 2 h produced no extra-corporeal occlusion, administering taprostene alone for 5 h, some clots did occur after 3–5 h, which caused premature termination of HD or made reinfusion impossible after 5 h (fig. 2). When 25 ng/kg/min was applied together with a continuous low-dose heparin for 5 h, only small clots were observed which did not impede HD or reinfusion.

When this dose was increased to 35 ng/kg/min, the small clots were still observed and all 5 patients experienced nausea and headaches during or after HD. No cardiovascular side effects were found.

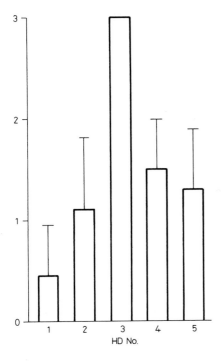

Fig. 2. Clot formation in the extracorporeal system (mean ± SD) during the 5 different dialysis regimens of the study design. Stages of clot formation: 0 = none, 1 = slight, 2 = large (but no premature termination of dialysis and partial reinfusion possible), 3 = complete.

Discussion

At the beginning of HD there is slight thrombopenia and stronger leukopenia, induced by the Cuprophan of the dialyzer membrane; these effects are no longer present 60 min after commencing HD [3, 4]. Cuprophan causes activation of complement, which in turn causes deposits of leukocyte aggregates in the pulmonary lymph vessels [5]. The slight initial thrombopenia has no connection with heparin-induced thrombopenia, but is likewise induced by the Cuprophan, due to thrombocytes adhering to the membrane [6]. Consequently, there is no difference between HD using solely heparin and HD using solely taprostene as regards leukopenia and thrombopenia.

On considering our design, it will first be clear that HD with PGI_2 reported as successful for 2 h [3] cannot be extended to 5 h, since during the 3rd to 5th h of HD the hypercoagulability continues progressively to increase and necessarily leads to massive formation of clots. However, the additional administration of a low-dose heparin [7] also seems to inhibit the plasmatic coagulation, so that only smaller clots occur which do not impede HD. These results are confirmed by the study of Rylance et al. [4], who, under the combination of PGI_2 and low-dose heparin, found statistically significant lower values of fibrinopeptide A than when giving PGI_2 alone.

Whereas taprostene is used for only 5 h in HD, it would need to be employed over a significantly longer period in the context of continuous hemofiltration (CH). On the basis of a case study of our group [8], in which taprostene was administered to a patient suffering from thrombotic thrombocytopenic purpura for 100 h without encountering any problems, and of other case studies reporting the use of PGI_2 in CH [9, 10], the use of taprostene in venovenous CH, in combination with a low-dose heparin and high blood flow rates, may be regarded as fundamentally practical. Although taprostene is less vasodilatory than PGI_2, it should not, however, be used in patients with arterial hypotension.

We also noted an extreme hyperfibrinogenemia (> 600 mg/dl) in a number of patients with a short hemofilter running time. In some of these cases, we used ancrod (Arvin®), the purified active fraction of the venom of the Malayan pit viper *Agkistrodon rhodostoma* for controlled defibrination [11, 12], reducing the fibrinogen concentration to 100–200 mg/dl and significantly increasing the hemofilter running time.

In general, there is a definite need for further systematic investigation of alternative antithrombotic management during CH, in the form of controlled multicenter trials.

References

1   Swartz RD, Flamenbaum W, Dubrow A, Hall JC, Crow JW, Cato A: Epoprostenol (PGI_2, prostacyclin) during high-risk hemodialysis: Preventing further bleeding complications. J Clin Pharmacol 1988;28:818–825.
2   Maurin N: Influence of platelet activity and red cell fluidity of epoprostenol and two stable prostacyclin analogues in vitro. Arzneimittelforsch/Drug Res 1986;36:1180–1183.
3   Turney JH, Williams LC, Fewell MR, Parsons V, Weston MJ: Platelet protection and heparin sparing with prostacyclin during regular dialysis therapy. Lancet 1980;ii:219–222.
4   Rylance PB, Gordge MP, Ireland H, Lane DA, Weston MJ: Haemodialysis with prostacyclin (epoprostenol) alone. Proc Eur Dial Transplant Assoc 1984;21:281–286.
5   Craddock PR, Fehr J, Brigham KL, Kronenberg RS, Jacobs HS: Complement and leukocyte-mediated pulmonary dysfunction in hemodialysis. N Engl J Med 1977;296:769–774.
6   Salzman EW: Role of platelets in blood-surface interactions. Fed Proc 1971;30:1503–1509.
7   Buccianti G, Pogliani E, Miradoli R, Colombi MA, Valenti G, Lorenz M, Polli EE: Reduction of plasma levels of betathromboglobulin and platelet factor 4 during hemodialysis: a possible role for a short acting inhibitor of platelet aggregation. Clin Nephrol 1982;18:204–208.

8   Maurin N, Glöckner WM, Sieberth HG: Treatment of a case of thrombotic thrombocy-
     topenic purpura (TTP) by plasma exchange and long-term infusion of the stable
     prostacyclin analogue taprostene. Thromb Haemost 1989;62:245.
9   Wendon J, Smithies M, Sheppard M, Bullen K, Tinker J, Bihari D: Continuous high
     volume venous–venous haemofiltration in acute renal failure. Intensive Care Med
     1989;15:358–363.
10   Zobel G, Ring E, Müller W: Continuous arteriovenous hemofiltration in premature
     infants. Crit Care Med 1989;17:534–536.
11   Roy J, Guidoin R, Martin L, Lephat H, Blais P, Marois M, Gagnon D, Awad J:
     Defibrinogenation as an alternative to heparinization in prolonged extracorporeal
     circulation. Res Exp Med 1980;176:219–234.
12   Zulys VJ, Teasdale SJ, Michel ER, Skala RA, Keating SE, Viger JR, Glynn MXF:
     Ancrod (Arvin®) as an alternative to heparin anticoagulation for cardiopulmonary
     bypass. Anesthesiology 1989;71:870–877.

Norbert Maurin, MD, Medical Clinic II, University Hospital Aachen,
Pauwelsstrasse 30, D–W–5100 Aachen (FRG)

Sieberth HG, Mann H, Stummvoll HK (eds): Continuous Hemofiltration.
Contrib Nephrol. Basel, Karger, 1991, vol 93, pp 210–214

Regional Citrate Anticoagulation for Continuous Arteriovenous Hemodialysis

An Update after 12 Months

Ravindra L. Mehta, Brian R. McDonald, David M. Ward[1]

University of California, San Diego UCSD Medical Center, San Diego, Calif., USA

Continuous arterioverious hemodialysis (CAVHD) is increasingly used as therapy for intensive-care unit (ICU) patients with acute renal failure (ARF) [1, 2]. Systemic anticoagulation with heparin (HEP-CAVHD) can increase risks of bleeding and thrombocytopenia. We previously described regional citrate anticoagulation for CAVHD (CIT-CAVHD) [3]; this paper reports further experience with this technique.

Patients and Methods

From December 1988 through March 1990, 34 ICU patients with ARF at the University of California San Diego (UCSD) Medical Center were treated with CAVHD. 23 patients received CIT-CAVHD, 12 received heparin initially (3 switched to CIT-CAVHD because of heparin-induced thrombocytopenia and 2 due to life-threatening bleeding) and 2 had saline flushes alone. 1 pediatric patient on HEP-CAVHD was excluded from analysis as he was on a pumped ECMO circuit. Similarly, both patients on saline flushes had filter life of <24 h and were not included. We retrospectively reviewed the method of anticoagulation used to maintain CAVHD filter patency. The CAVHD technique, anticoagulation, blood sampling, monitoring, calculations and statistical analysis were described in detail previously [3]. A schematic diagram of the circuit used is shown in figure 1.

Results

Clinical Features. 24 patients were on the surgical and 10 on the medical service. 17% of patients undergoing CIT-CAVHD and 25% undergoing HEP-CAVHD had liver failure. Anticoagulation selection was based on clinical criteria; patients with high bleeding risk received citrate or saline flushes. 11 patients received HEP-CAVHD; CIT-CAVHD only was

---

[1] We thank Maria Pascual, Petrea Monson and L. Taylor-Donald for their contributions.

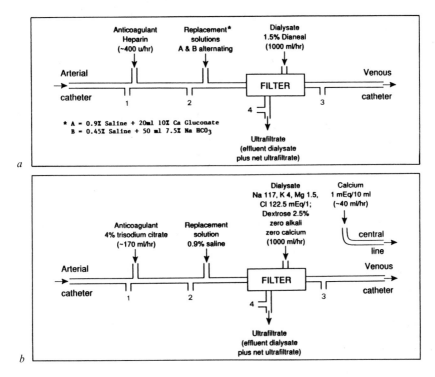

Fig. 1. Comparison of circuit diagrams for HEP-CAVHD (*a*) and CIT-CAVHD (*b*). Sampling ports are marked: 1 = peripheral; 2 = prefilter; 3 = postfilter; 4 = ultrafiltrate. (This figure is reprinted from Mehta et al. [3], with permission from Springer, Berlin).

used in 20 patients and replaced HEP-CAVHD in another 3. All were critically ill, fluid overloaded and ventilator-dependent at initiation of CAVHD. 9 survived and 7 regained renal function. 2 required intermittent hemodialysis after stabilizing on CAVHD and subsequently expired. Of the 26 who died, 9 had irreversible brain damage and 3 succumbed to hepatic encephalopathy.

Technical Adequacy. Fluid and electrolyte balance was achieved in all patients. Table 1 depicts the sieving coefficient for blood urea nitrogen (BUN) mean blood flow rates, ultrafiltration rate (UFR), convective and diffusive BUN clearance, and total clearances for the heparin versus citrate group. Mean blood flow rates were not different in either group. UFRs ranged from 4.8 to 20 ml/min and were significantly higher for the citrate group (p = 0.005). Dialyzer urea clearances ranged from 9 to 25.9 ml/min for HEP-CAVHD (mean 19.9 ml/min) and from 12 to 32.5 ml/min for

Table 1. Filter efficacy in heparin versus citrate CAVHD

Group	SC	BFR ml/mm	UFR ml/mm	BUN clearance, ml/min		Total Cl ml/min
				convective	diffusive	
Heparin	0.78 (0.02)	83.5 (6.4)	8.57 (0.52)	6.79 (0.56)	13.1 (0.55)	19.76 (1.04)
Citrate	0.86 (0.014)[a]	94.23 (4.95)[b]	10.52 (0.42)[c]	9.14 (0.39)[d]	14.38 (0.24)[e]	23.5 (0.53)[f]

Results are means with SEM in parentheses. SC = Sieving coefficient; BFR = blood flow rate; Cl = clearance. Citrate versus heparin: [a]$p = 0.044$; [b]$p = 0.192$; [c]$p = 0.005$; [d]$p = 0.001$; [e]$p = 0.032$; [f]$p = 0.003$.

CIT-CAVHD (mean 23.5 ml/min, $p = 0.003$). BUN sieving coefficients were higher for CIT-CAVHD as compared to HEP-CAVHD ($p = 0.044$).

Anticoagulation Adequacy. Both groups had adequate anticoagulation as evidenced by activated clotting time (ACT) and partial thromboplastin time determinations. Baseline ACT values were determined in all patients prior to anticoagulation. Peripheral ACT determinations done periodically during CAVHD revealed a tendency toward progressive elevation with heparin and no elevation with citrate infusion. A total of 4,804 h of CAVHD was done in 31 patients, utilizing 83 filters. The mean filter life for CIT-CAVHD was superior to HEP-CAVHD but was not statistically significant ($p = 0.07$; table 2). Comparing the median filter lifetimes by life table analysis showed that the citrate and heparin groups had similar results ($p = 0.09$). When all filters were considered, 72-hour patency was 40% for CIT-CAVHD versus 25% for HEP-CAVHD filters. Overall, 38.6% of filters were changed due to clotting, 14.5% due to decreased efficacy, 25.3% were electively discontinued, 15.7% because of the patient's death and 4.8% due to access-related problems. More HEP-CAVHD filters clotted than did CIT-CAVHD filters (50 vs. 34.5%) and more had decreased efficacy (22.7 vs. 11.5%); however, these were not statistically significant.

Complications of Treatment. CIT- and HEP-CAVHD complications are shown in table 3. Access-related problems included hematoma at the catheter insertion site in the femoral vein, peripheral ischemia from a large bore catheter in the pediatric patient (citrate group) and localized hematomas in the heparin group. Serum total and ionized calcium levels were monitored in all CIT-CAVHD patients. Peripheral ionized calcium levels ranged from 0.84 to 1.24 mmol/l in most patients. No patient developed symptomatic hypocalcemia. There was no evidence for electrocardiographic

Table 2. CAVHD at UCSD (December 88–March 90): Anticoagulant method and filter patency

Group	Number of patients	Total hours of CAVHD	Total number of filters	Average life of filters, h (mean ± SEM)[a]
All	31	4,804	83	57.9 ± 4.7
Heparin	11	1,018	23	44.3 ± 6.1
Citrate	23	2,886	61	63.1 ± 5.9

[a] ANOVA heparin vs. citrate: p = 0.07.

Table 3. Complications related to CAVHD

Group	Number of patients	Total hours of CAVHD	Access related	Bleeding	Thrombo-cytopenia	Metabolic alkalosis
All	31	4,804	4 (12.9)	3 (9.7)	1 (3.2)	6 (19.36)
Heparin	11	1,018	2 (18)	3 (27)	1 (9)	0
Citrate	23	2,886	2 (6)	0	0	6 (26.1)

Results are numbers of patients with percentages in parentheses.

changes or myocardial depression. Peripheral serum citrate levels ranged from 0.074 to 3.71 mmol/l. Transient metabolic alkalosis developed in 6 patients and was easily corrected by infusion of 0.2 M HCl through a central vein. CIT-CAVHD was continued during surgery and anesthesia without problems. Hypernatremia was seen only in 1 patient while the CIT-CAVHD protocol was being developed.

Discussion

CAVHD is used in critically ill patients at high risk of death or major complications. Our regional citrate anticoagulation protocol provides an alternative to systemic heparin anticoagulation. The experience we now report is extensive and shows that the technique is safe, practical and particularly useful for high-risk cases.

We modified the original CAVHD method developed by Geronemus [4] by routinely incorporating prefilter replacement solution and maintaining the UFR at approximately 7–10 ml/min, thus influencing convective clearance. The zero calcium, zero alkali dialysate permits removal of calcium-citrate chelate and allows regional anticoagulation with citrate with no significant metabolic problems. A hyponatremic dialysate allows removal of the sodium load imposed by the trisodium citrate. CIT-CAVHD allows adequate anticoagulation as evidenced by filter patency rates equal to or greater than with HEP-CAVHD. The better clearances associated with CIT-CAVHD may reflect the enhanced convective clearance produced by adding citrate before filter. CIT-CAVHD was well tolerated by most patients, including those with hepatic insufficiency who metabolized citrate despite significant deterioration in liver function. Citrate flow rate was adjusted based on postfilter ACTs and minimal alteration in anticoagulation status was seen.

The incidence of bleeding complications with even low-dose systemic heparinization can be as high as 30% [5–7] and is comparable to our experience. CIT-CAVHD avoids this and heparin-induced thrombocytopenia. The trade-offs of citrate versus heparin are increased complexity of the citrate procedure and higher risk of metabolic alkalosis in patients. However, with careful and close monitoring, nurses can easily perform the procedure and metabolic alkalosis can be minimized by adjusting citrate flow rates depending on the blood flow rates. Our experience demonstrates that regional anticoagulation with citrate offers a practical alternative to systemic anticoagulation with heparin for CAVHD. When properly monitored, volume and solute balance can be effectively achieved in the ICU setting. This citrate anticoagulation protocol should also be applicable to pumped systems, such as continuous venovenous hemodialysis.

References

1   Gibney RTN, Stollery DE, Lefebvre RE, et al: Continuous arteriovenous hemodialysis: An alternative therapy for acute renal failure associated with critical illness. Can Med Assoc 1988;139:861–866.

2   Schneider NS, Geronemus RP: Continuous arteriovenous hemodialysis. Kidney Int 1988;5:159–162.

3   Mehta RL, McDonald BR, Aguilar M, Ward DM: Regional citrate anticoagulation for continuous arteriovenous hemodialysis in critically ill patients. Kidney Int 1990; 38:976–981.

4   Geronemus RP: Slow continuous hemodialysis. Trans Am Soc Artif Intern Organs 1988; 24:59–60.

5   Pinnick RV, Wiegmann TB, Diederich DA: Regional citrate anticoagulation for hemodialysis in the patient at high risk for bleeding. N Engl J Med 1983;308:258–263.

6   Flanigan MJ, Von Brecht JV, Freeman RM, Lim VS: Reducing the hemorrhagic complications of hemodialysis: A controlled comparison of low-dose heparin and citrate anticoagulation. Am J Kidney Dis 1987;9:147–153.

7   Lauer A, Sacaggi A, Ronco C, et al: Continuous arteriovenous hemofiltration in the critically ill patient. Ann Intern Med 1983;99:455.

Dr. Ravindra L. Mehta, University of California, San Diego, UCSD Medical Center, 225 Dickinson, San Diego, CA 92103 (USA)

Sieberth HG, Mann H, Stummvoll HK (eds): Continuous Hemofiltration.
Contrib Nephrol. Basel, Karger, 1991, vol 93, pp 215–217

Nafamostat Mesylate as Anticoagulant in Continuous Hemofiltration and Continuous Hemodiafiltration

Yoshio Ohtake, Hiroyuki Hirasawa, Takao Sugai, Shigeto Oda,
Hidetoshi Shiga, Kenichi Matsuda, Nobuya Kitamura

Department of Emergency and Critical Care Medicine, Chiba University School of
Medicine, Chiba, Japan

Continuous hemofiltration (CHF) and continuous hemodiafiltration (CHDF) have become important therapeutic tools in the anuric critically ill patient. However, the bleeding complication caused with anticoagulant is a serious complication of CHF and CHDF. The present study was undetaken to elucidate the relationship between various anticoagulants and the incidences of bleeding complication during CHF and CHDF and to decide the optimal dose of the anticoagulants.

Material and Methods

Forty-three critically ill patients, on whom CHF and/or CHDF were performed for at least 48 h between October 1985 and July 1990, entered the study. Heparin, low molecular weight heparin (LMWH) [1] and nafamostat mesylate (NM) [2] were used as anticoagulant during CHF and CHDF and bleeding incidences were studied. Activated coagulation time (ACT) [3] was applied as a monitoring to decide the optimal dose of anticoagulants. The correlations between ACT and dose of anticoagulants were studied. The concentrations of NM in artery and extracorporeal circulation were measured.

Results

The bleeding incidences with heparin, LMWH and NM during CHF and/or CHDF, were 67, 29 and 4%, respectively. The dose of NM showed significant positive correlation with ACT. On the other hand, the dose of heparin and LMWH did not correlate with ACT. In addition, there is no correlation between ACT and dose of heparin among the patients with bleeding complication during CHF. This indicates that bleeding complication develops even with a low dose of heparin. The optimal dose of LMWH seems to be less than 2.5 U/kg/h. Our past experiences let us

Table 1. Anticoagulants for CHF and CHDF

	Heparin	Low molecular weight heparin	Nafamostat mesylate
Mechanism of action	inhibition of thrombin, IXa, Xa, XIa, XIIa with ATIII	inhibition of Xa	inhibition of thrombin, Xa, XIIa, prohibition of platelet aggregation
Half-life time	90 min	180 min	5–8 min
Optimal dose		<2.5 U/kg/h	0.1 mg/kg/h
Monitoring	ACT	anti-Xa activity	ACT
Bleeding incidence	8/12 (67%)	5/17 (29%)	1/23 (4%)

conclude that the optimal ACT is around 150 s during blood purification. Getting 150 s of ACT, NM is needed in a dose 0.1 mg/kg/h.

The concentrations of NM in arterial blood is 163 ± 88 ng/ml. On the other hand, the concentrations in blood immediately below the infusion line of NM is $4,420 \pm 1,671$ ng/ml and that in blood of inlet of flexible double lumen catheter is $2,921 \pm 450$ ng/ml. In addition, there is significant correlation between ACT and concentration of NM.

Discussion

When we use anticoagulants, deciding the optimal dose is very important to avoid not only bleeding but also coagulation within the blood circuit. ACT has been widely used to decide the optimal dose of heparin during extracorporeal circulation in cardiovascular surgery and HD [3]. However, our results indicate that there is no significant correlation between ACT and dose of heparin during CHD and/or CHDF (table 1). In addition, bleeding complication develops even with low dose heparin. The reasons why heparin causes bleeding complication are that since half-life time of heparin is about 90 min, it accumulates during CHF, and that metabolism of heparin is delayed due to hepatic failure which sometimes complicates to anuric critically ill patients. Therefore, it is indicated that heparin should be avoided to use as anticoagulant during CHF.

LMWH has been reported to cause less bleeding complication than hepain dose [1]. Our study also indicated that there was a significant difference in bleeding incidences between heparin and LMWH. However, bleeding complication still developed in 29% of the patients with LMWH. When we use LMWH during CHF and CHDF, it gives us two problems: one is that no bedside monitoring is available to decide the optimal dose, and the other is the longer half-time than that of heparin. For the above reasons, heparin and LMWH are not excellent anticoagulants for CHF and CHDF.

NM is one of protease inhibitors which also has some pharmacological actions on the coagulation system [2]. Its half-time is 5–8 min which makes NM a suitable anticoagulant during extracorporeal circulation. Considering suitable life time and the availability of bedside monitoring in addition to low bleeding incidence, NM is the anticoagulant of first choice in anuric critically ill patients.

References

1   Holmer E, Mattsson C, Nilsson S: Anticoagulant and antithrombotic effects of heparin and low molecular weight heparin fragments in rabbits. Thromb Res 1982;25:475–485.
2   Ohtake Y, Hirasawa H, Sugai T, Oda S, Shiga H, Matsuda K, Kitamura N, Odaka M, Tabata Y: A study on anticoagulants in continuous hemofiltration (CHF). Jpn J Artif Organs 1990;19:744–748.
3   Bull BS, Korpman RA, Huse WM, Briggs BD: Heparin therapy during extracorporeal circulation. I. Problems inherent in existing heparin protocols. J Thorac Cardiovasc Surg 1975;69:674–684.

Dr. Y. Ohtake, Department of Emergency and Critical Care Medicine,
Chiba University School of Medicine, 1–8–1 Inohana, Chiba 280 (Japan)

Sieberth HG, Mann H, Stummvoll HK (eds): Continuous Hemofiltration.
Contrib Nephrol. Basel, Karger, 1991, vol 93, pp 218–220

Use of Prostacyclin as the Only Anticoagulant during Continuous Venovenous Hemofiltration

Rafael Ponikvar, Aljoša Kandus, Jadranka Buturović, Rado Kveder

Department of Nephrology, University Medical Center, Ljubljana, Yugoslavia

Prostacyclin (PGI$_2$), discovered by J. Vane in 1976, was in the late seventies for the first time applied as anticoagulant (antiaggregating) drug for hemodialysis, charcoal hemoperfusion and cardiopulmonary bypass operations. PGI$_2$ is a potent vasodilator and the most potent inhibitor of platelet aggregation yet discovered. It is normally produced by vascular tissues of humans, half-life is about 2 min and the effect on platelets disappears 30 min after the cessation of intravenous administration. PGI$_2$ has systemic effects and is not inactivated in the lungs. Systemic vasodilation produces hypotension which is dose dependent. PGI$_2$ was advised to be used instead of heparin during extracorporeal procedures in patients who were at risk of bleeding [1].

The aim of this prospective clinical study was to evaluate the influence of PGI$_2$ on some hemostatic parameters and on circulatory stability of the patients with acute renal failure (ARF) and multiorgan failure treated with continuous venovenous hemofiltration (CVVH).

Materials and Methods

Seven patients with ARF and multiorgan failure, 5 women and 2 men, aged 33–59 years (mean 47 ± 9.9) were treated with CVVH and PGI$_2$ as the sole anticoagulant. The main causes of ARF were septicemia in 4 patients, polytrauma in 1, Wegener's granulomatosis in 1 and heart failure with ventricular septum defect (VSD) in 1 patient. Six of them required mechanical ventilation and were at risk of bleeding. Amicon 20 (Amicon Division of Grace AG, Lausanne, Switzerland) and Bellco BL 621 and BL 627 hemofilters (Bellco, Mirandola, Italy) with polysulfone membrane were used. A blood pump from hemodialysis monitor Gambro AK-10 was used (Gambro, Lund, Sweden). Hemodialysis catheters placed into femoral veins were used as vascular access (Deseret Medical Inc., Sundy, Utah, USA). Flolan (PGI$_2$) (Wellcome Foundation, London, UK) was infused in a continuous infusion at a dose of 5 ng/kg/min. Infusion started 15 min before the beginning of the CVVH procedures. Hemofiltration solution Baxter HF-5, containing lactate (Baxter SpA, Rome, Italy) was infused postdilutionally. Systolic (SBP) and diastolic (DBP) blood pressures and heart rate

Table 1. SBP, DBP, HR, platelet count, PTT, PT and serum fibrinogen during CVVH with PGI$_2$

	Hours				
	0	6	12	18	24
SBP, mm Hg	110 ± 32	119 ± 26	119 ± 27	108 ± 28	105 ± 27
DBP, mm Hg	61 ± 23	65 ± 20	71 ± 20	64 ± 20	60 ± 24
HR, beats/min	111 ± 23	116 ± 29	105 ± 18	116 ± 31	123 ± 21
Platelet count × 10/l	107 ± 55	110 ± 84	114 ± 62	127 ± 79	109 ± 72
PTT, s	60.3 ± 39.8	59.8 ± 42.6	44.0 ± 8.6	35.4 ± 3.8	42.5 ± 2.1
PT, 1 = 100%	0.48 ± 0.17	0.51 ± 0.24	0.52 ± 0.22	0.47 ± 0.20	0.50 ± 0.23
Fibrinogen, g/l	4 ± 0.9	4 ± 1.6	4 ± 1.3	3.8 ± 0.8	4 ± 1.6

(HR) were measured hourly till the end of the treatment. Serum concentrations of creatinine, urea and fibrinogen, platelet count, partial thromboplastin time (PTT) and prothrombin time (PT) were measured at the beginning and every 6 h of the treatment.

Results

CVVH treatment lasted from 13 to 360 h (mean 90 ± 131). Mean blood flow was 155 ± 70 ml/min, ultrafiltration rate 1,425 ± 354 ml/h and ultrafiltration 156 ± 107 ml/h. Lifespan of hemofilters was 13–48 h (mean 19.7). A total of 630 h of CVVH with PGI$_2$ was performed. Serum concentration of creatinine diminished by about 30% in 24 h (serum creatinine at the beginning 488 ± 170, after 24 h 337 ± 147 μmol/l). Serum urea concentration decreased from 43.7 ± 10.7 to 31.5 ± 10.3 mmol/l in 24 h. SBP, DBP, HR, platelet count, PTT, PT, and serum concentration of fibrinogen for the first day of treatment are presented in table 1. Three of 6 patients with ARF and multiorgan failure survived. Renal function of the patient with ARF and heart failure with VSD improved within the first day of treatment.

Discussion

PGI$_2$ at a dose of 5 ng/kg/min, which was usually used during hemodialysis, was safely applied during CVVH treatment in patients with ARF and multiorgan failure. Circulatory instability was not observed and CVVH procedures did not have to be discontinued because of profound fall of blood pressure [2]. Platelet count did not change during CVVH. There was no influence of PGI$_2$ on the intrinsic and extrinsic coagulation system. According to our experiences with CVVH with heparin, lifespan of hemofilters in CVVH with PGI$_2$ was about 30% shorter. Although 6/7 patients were at high risk of hemorrhage, there was no excessive bleeding during CVVH. PGI_2 seems to be a useful anticoagulant drug in the treatment of severe ill and hypotensive patients with risk of hemorrhage. Its use might be even more desirable if the cytoprotective effect and improvement of tissue oxygenation by PGI_2 were to be unequivocally proven [3]. Three of 6 patients with multiorgan failure survived probably because of good medical treatment. The possible role of PGI_2 in the improving of the survival rate of patients with multiorgan failure needs further investigation.

References

1   Vane JR: The discovery of prostacyclin: in Williams EB (ed): Prostacyclin, Past, Present and Future. Current Clinical Concepts. London, The Wellcome Foundation, 1985, No 3, pp 7–16.
2   Miller LC, Hall JC, Crown JW, Cato AE, Edson JR, Scheinman JI: Hemodialysis in heparin-associated thrombocytopenia: Epoprostenol (PGI_2) as sole anticoagulant. Dial Transplant 1985;14:579–580.
3   Bihari D, Smithies M: The pathogenesis of multiple organ failure associated with septicaemic shock; in Williams EB (ed): Prostacyclin, Past, Present and Future. Current Clinical Concepts. London, The Wellcome Foundation, 1985, No 3, pp 49–59.

Rafael Ponikvar, MD, Department of Nephrology, University Medical Center, Zaloška 7, YU–61000 Ljubljana (Yugoslavia)

Sieberth HG, Mann H, Stummvoll HK (eds): Continuous Hemofiltration.
Contrib Nephrol. Basel, Karger, 1991, vol 93, pp 221–224

Guidelines to the Use of Enoxaparin in Slow Continuous Hemodialysis

A. Wynckel[a], *B. Bernieh*[a], *O. Toupance*[a], *P.H. N'Guyen*[b], *T. Wong*[a], *S. Lavaud*[a], *J. Chanard*[a]

[a]Service de Néphrologie et [b]Laboratoire d'Hématologie, Centre Hospitalier Universitaire, Reims, France

Anticoagulation which is necessary for slow continuous hemodialysis (SCH) can lead to complications in critically ill patients. Low-molecular-weight heparins (LMWH) are not being used successfully in conventional hemodialysis [1, 2]. Moreover, when LMWH are tested over a long period in randomized trials patients require fewer erythrocyte transfusions [1]. The aim of the study was to evaluate an LMWH, namely enoxaparin (Lovenox®), in SCH. Enoxaparin [3] is an LMWH (4.5 – 5 kilodaltons) which is characterized by a mean anti-Xa activity of 113 IU/mg and an anti-Xa/anti-IIa ratio higher than 4.

Patients and Methods

7 patients with multiorgan failure (mean simplified acute physiology score = 16.15 ± 6.45) and requiring SCH were included into the study. All received amine pressive agents. Patients who needed heparinization for any thrombotic event or who were hemodialyzed for less than 24 h were excluded. Initial thrombocyte count was less than $50 \times 10^9/l$ in 5 patients.

Vascular access used a Scribner shunt in 1 patient and a double-lumen venous catheter with a BSM22 blood system (Hospal) in 6 patients. An AN69S parallel-plate dialyzer ($0.5 \, m^2$) was used and ideally changed every day (n = 29, mean duration 22.75 ± 5.70 h). The blood and dialysate flow rates ranged from 60 to 80 ml/min and from 16 to 33 ml/min, respectively.

In order to define adequate anticoagulation during SCH, optimal doses of enoxaparin were estimated from results obtained in intermittent hemodialysis. A mean anti-Xa activity higher than 0.25 IU/ml measured at the end of the procedure was necessary to prevent thrombosis.

The following regimen was tested: initial pulse of 40 mg, then intermittent administration of doses between 10 and 40 mg every 6 h, in order to maintain trough anti-Xa activity between 0.25 and 0.50 IU/ml.

Anti-Xa activity was measured with a chromogenic substrate (CBS 3139, Stago, France). Activated partial thromboplastin time (APTT) was simultaneously monitored with a commercially available assay (General Diagnostics). Blood samples were drawn every 6 h.

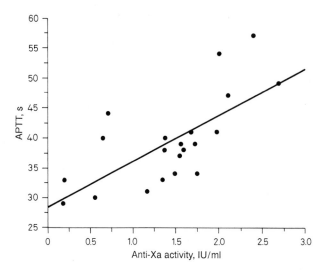

Fig. 1. SCH and enoxaparin correlation between anti-Xa activity and APTT in 2 patients with normal initial APTT (y = 7.7 x + 28.4; r = 0.693; p = 0.0005).

Results

4 patients died from causes not related to the SCH technique. No bleeding complications nor a decrease in thrombocyte count were observed. SCH was efficient to treat acute renal failure. Urea clearance was 90% of dialysate flow (p < 0.001).

In 6 patients anti-Xa activity was 0.47 ± 0.10 IU/ml (n = 46). These results were obtained with a daily dose of 1.86 ± 0.75 mg/kg. In an additional patient, anti-Xa activity was 3 times higher. However, it did not improve SCH performances nor induce bleeding.

A positive correlation was found between anti-Xa activity and APTT in patients with normal initial APTT as well as in patients with prolonged APTT (fig. 1, 2). Clotting of the extracorporeal circuit was noted in 2 cases where anti-Xa activity was 0.14 and 0.18 IU/ml, respectively.

Discussion

These results suggest that enoxaparin is efficient to handle SCH. Dialysis efficiency was quite similar to that previously obtained with unfractionated heparin [4] where urea clearance was equal to dialysate flow rate.

The mechanism of the antithrombotic effect of LMWH is still controversial. Antithrombin activity may be essential to the antithrombotic and anticoagulant effect: thrombin induces fibrin formation and can activate

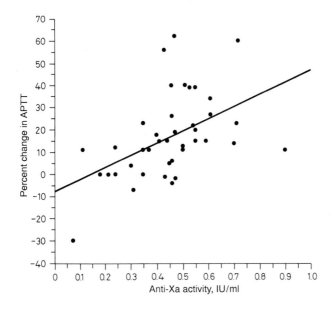

Fig. 2. SCH and enoxaparin correlation between anti-Xa activity and percent changes in APTT in 5 patients with abnormal APTT before starting therapy. (y = 54.9 x − 7.8; r = 0.50; p = 0.0013).

factor V and factor VIII. However, anti-Xa activity plays a role. Lane et al. [5] found a negative relationship between anti-Xa activity and fibrinopeptide A level during hemodialysis for chronic renal failure. Measurement of anti-Xa activity is probably insufficient but largely reflects the antithrombotic effect of LMWH. Even at optimal anti-Xa activity levels does LMWH increase APTT. Therefore, LMWH administration implies precise biological monitoring. Nevertheless, accidental bleeding was not observed in this study.

In conclusion, enoxaparin is a suitable LMWH for SCH. A trough anti-Xa activity between 0.25 and 0.50 IU/ml can prevent clotting without side effects.

References

1   Schrader J, Stibbe W, Armstrong VW, Kandt M, Muche R, Köstering H, Seidel D, Scheler F: Comparison of low molecular weight heparin to standard heparin in hemodialysis/hemofiltration. Kidney Int 1988;33:890–896.
2   Dechelette E, Pouzol P, Jurkovitz C, Kuentz F, Polack B, Cuzin E: Utilisation de l'énoxaparine pour l'anticoagulation du circuit extracorporel des hémodialyses à haut risque hémorragique. J Mal Vasc 1987;12:105–107.

3   Vinazzer H, Woler M: A new low molecular weight heparin fragment (PK 10169): In vitro and in vivo studies. Thromb Res 1985;40:135–146.

4   Wynckel A, Toupance O, Melin J-P, Lavaud S, Wong T, Chanard J: L'hémodialyse continue à bas débit sanguin et à bas débit de dialysat dans le traitement de l'insuffisance rénale aiguë. Néphrologie, 1990;11:123–127.

5   Lane DA, Flynn A, Ireland H, Anastassiades E, Curtis JR: On the evaluation of heparin and low molecular weight heparin in haemodialysis for chronic renal failure. Haemostasis 1986;16(suppl 2):38–47.

Dr. A. Wynckel, Service de Néphrologie, Hôpital Maison Blanche, 45, rue Cognacq-Jay, F–51000 Reims (France)

Miscellaneous

Sieberth HG, Mann H, Stummvoll HK (eds): Continuous Hemofiltration.
Contrib Nephrol. Basel, Karger, 1991, vol 93, pp 225–233

Continuous vs. Intermittent Forms of Haemofiltration and/or Dialysis in the Management of Acute Renal Failure in Patients with Defective Cerebral Autoregulation at Risk of Cerebral Oedema

A. Davenport, E.J. Will, A.M. Davison

Department of Renal Medicine, St. James's University Hospital, Leeds, UK

Patients with chronic renal failure have been reported to develop cerebral oedema as a consequence of treatment with conventional haemodialysis [1]. This has been confirmed by studies using computerised cerebral tomographic [2] and nuclear magnetic resonance scanning techniques [3]. Symptoms, fortunately, are usually minimal but occasionally nausea, vomiting, blurring of vision and even fits may occur [4]. Major symptoms are usually confined to patients with structural brain lesions or an abnormal blood brain barrier, as reported in severe malaria or leptospirosis [5].

Patients who develop fulminant hepatic failure (FHF) are at risk of dying from cerebral oedema [6]. Patients who in addition develop acute renal failure have been shown to have an increased mortality [7], due to cerebral oedema. This has been reported to be more difficult to control than in patients with hepatic failure alone [8]. This is due to a combination of the development of both cytotoxic and vasogenic cerebral oedema (fig. 1).

We studied the effect of different renal replacement modalities on intracranial pressure (ICP) in a group of patients with both acute hepatic and renal failure. As this group were at risk of developing cerebral oedema we wished to investigate whether different types of dialysis treatments would affect ICP to account for the failure of previous studies to show improved survival on standard haemodialysis treatment [10]. In the absence of clear evidence we felt justified to explore the hypothesis that intermittent and continuous treatments were equally effective in acute hepatorenal failure.

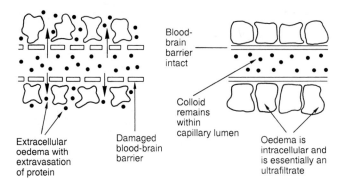

Fig. 1. Schematic diagram to show the basic differences between the pathogenesis of cytotoxic (right) and vasogenic (left) cerebral oedema.

Patients and Methods

Patients. Twenty-two patients who had developed grade IV hepatic coma following paracetamol (acetaminophen) self-poisoning and oliguric renal failure were studied. The group comprised 14 males, 8 females, median age 30 years (range 21–62), urine output < 10 ml/h, median serum creatinine 570 μmol/l (range 378–834). All patients were treated with elective hyperventilation (PaCO$_2$ less than 4.5 kPa, 33 mm Hg), sedated with propofol, median dose 100 mg/h (range 50–200), paralysed with atracurium, median dose 1 mg/h (range 0.5–2.0) and given the analgesic alfentanyl, median dose 1 mg/h (range 0.5–2.0). In addition, all patients were nursed with the head of the bed raised upwards by 10–20°.

Methods. Patients were initially randomised to receive either daily intermittent machine haemofiltration (MHF) or continuous treatment using either spontaneous arteriovenous haemofiltration (CAVHF) or haemofiltration with dialysis (CAVHD). All treatments were designed to be isovolaemic to exclude changes in intravascular volume. MHF was carried out using a haemofiltration machine (Gambro AB, Lund, Sweden) a Gambro FH77 haemofilter, blood pump speed 200 ml/min, transmembrane pressure 200 mm Hg, and a 17-litre exchange of fluid taking on average 4 h. CAVHF/CAVHD was through a flat plate haemofilter (Hospal 2400, Rhone-Poulenc, Lyons, France), with an ultrafiltration rate varying between 400 and 1,600 ml/h. The same haemofiltration substitution fluid/dialysate was used in all treatments (Pharmacia, Uppsala, Sweden), with a sodium concentration of 140 mmol/l. During CAVHD the dialysate flow was 16.6 ml/min. If anticoagulation was deemed necessary, heparin was infused to maintain whole blood clotting times between 100 and 120 s (using a thrombotest reaction). Prior to commencing treatment the pulmonary artery wedge pressure was recorded and 5% human albumin solution administered if the patient was found to be hypovolaemic, pulmonary artery wedge pressure of 9 mm Hg or less.

Measurements. ICP was monitored using a subdural catheter which had been aseptically inserted through a frontal burr hole in an adjacent operating theatre. Radial arterial blood pressure was recorded and the cerebral perfusion pressure derived from the difference between the ICP measured with respect to the frontal burr hole and the mean arterial blood pressure recorded at the carotid bifurcation. Cardiac output was measured using a room temperature thermodilution method. All pressures were transduced (Gould P10 Ez, Spectromed, Ill., USA) and both continuously displayed and recorded (Mennen Horizon, Mennen Medical, Buffalo, N.Y., USA). During treatment with the various modes of renal replacement therapy, ICP was treated if greater than 20 mm Hg and the cerebral perfusion pressure supported if less than 50 mm Hg.

Statistical Analysis. Intragroup analysis was performed using either the Wilcoxon rank sum pair test or the paired t test and intergroup analysis by either the Mann-Whitney U test or by Student's t test. Statistical significance was taken at or below the 5% level.

Results

There were no differences in conventional liver function tests between those treated by MHF and continuous techniques (CAVHF/D), mean prothrombin ratio 4.1 (range 3.6–7.1) vs. 7.9 (2.9–14.0) (normal < 1.1) and mean serum alanine transaminase 5,590 IU/l (1,540–41,300) vs. 7,900 IU/l (2,400–14,000) (normal < 35 IU/l), although the values tended to be greater in the CAVHF/D group.

Initially, patients were randomised to receive either MHF of CAVHF/D treatment; however, due to technical problems with the spontaneous circuits, some patients at rise of cerebral oedema were treated by both systems. These patients showed marked differences in the behaviour of ICP during the different modes of treatment (fig. 2). Following this observation and the rapid demise of 2 patients with increased ICP during MHF, a new policy was adopted, whereby all patients thought to be at imminent risk of dying from cerebral oedema were treated by continuous techniques.

In total ICP was recorded during 50 MHF treatments, and the first 5 h of 18 CAVHF and 10 CAVHD treatments. During 206 h of MHF treatment mannitol or sedative boluses were required on 36 occasions to control a sustained (ICP > 20 mm Hg lasting 5 min or longer and unrelated to nursing procedures, physiotherapy, etc.) increase in ICP, compared to 16 interventions during 570 h of CAVHF therapy (p < 0.01) and 27 interventions during 840 h of CAVHD (p < 0.05).

Due to the subsequent assignment of patients to different treatment modes, those treated by CAVHF/CAVHD had a significantly greater ICP at the start of treatment compared to those treated by MHF (fig. 3). During treatment with CAVHF/CAVHD the ICP remained stable, whereas during MHF treatment there was a significant increase. The greatest increase occurred during the first hour of treatment, when the change in serum osmolality was small from 316 ± 5 mosm/kg (mean ± SEM) to 314 ± 5 mosm/kg. Thereafter, ICP continued to increase and only declined after treatment had been completed (fig. 3). CAVHF treatment resulted in an initial small reduction in ICP of 3 ± 1% during the first hour of treatment compared to CAVHD where ICP remained stable.

The mean arterial blood pressure prior to treatment was lower in the

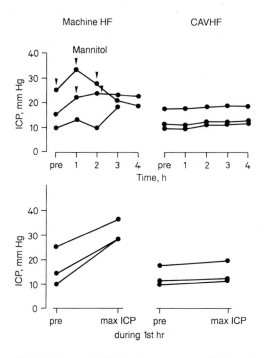

Fig. 2. Changes in ICP during treatment with intermittent machine haemofiltration and CAVHF in the same patient.

CAVHF/CAVHD group prior to treatment, 74 ± 4 mm Hg, compared to the MHF-treated group, 82 ± 4 mm Hg, $p < 0.05$. During treatment there was a reduction in arterial blood pressure. Maximal reduction occurred during the first hour and levels did not return to the baseline value until MHF treatment had been completed. Mean arterial blood pressure did not significantly decline during the continuous techniques, although compared to CAVHF there was a $7 \pm 4\%$ reduction during the first hour of CAVHD treatment.

Basal cerebral perfusion pressure was lower in the continuously treated group, 59 ± 5 mm Hg, compared to the MHF group, 72 ± 5 mm Hg, $p < 0.05$. Although the cerebral perfusion pressure remained stable during the continuous therapies, it declined during MHF and did not return to the baseline values until treatment had ended. The maximum decline in perfusion pressure occurred during the first hour, to a value of 62 ± 4 mm Hg, $p < 0.01$. Compared to CAVHF, where cerebral perfusion pressure remained stable during the 1st hour of treatment, there was a small decrease of $6 \pm 3\%$ during CAVHD.

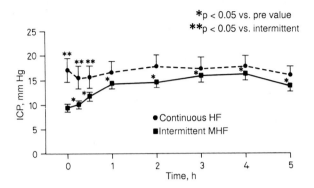

Fig. 3. The effect of treatment with daily intermittent machine haemofiltration and CAVHF/CAVHD on ICP. Mean values ± SEM.

Cardiac output remained stable during the continuous modes of treatment but declined during the first hour of MHF treatment (fig. 4). In addition to a consequent reduction in net tissue oxygen delivery there was also a reduction in tissue oxygen uptake, without any statistically significant increase in the tissue oxygen extraction ratio (fig. 4). Following termination of MHF there was an increase in cardiac output, net tissue oxygen delivery, tissue oxygen uptake and the oxygen extraction ratio, suggesting that a net tissue oxygen debt had developed during MHF.

Discussion

Patients with FHF have an abnormal circulatory state, as evidenced by an increased cardiac output and reduced systemic vascular resistance. Despite the increased cardiac output, shunting of blood occurs at the microcirculatory level resulting in tissue hypoxia [11]. This also occurs in the cerebral circulation [11] and results in damage to the blood-brain barrier [9]. In this study there was a correlation between the ICP and the mean arterial blood pressure (fig. 5) showing that for the majority of patients studied the normal mechanisms concerned in cerebral autoregulation were not functioning. Under these circumstances cerebral blood flow becomes dependent upon the cardiac output and the cerebral perfusion pressure. Cerebral hypoxia results in the release of local arteriolar vasodilators, such as adenosine, causing an increase in ICP [12].

Despite optimum positioning of the patient, the use of elective hyperventilation and propofol [13], the continuously treated group had an abnormally increased ICP prior to treatment (normal <10 mm Hg). These

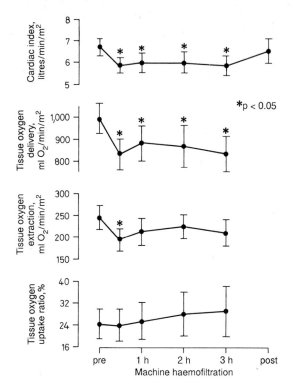

Fig. 4. Change in CI, tissue oxygen delivery (DO$_2$), tissue oxygen uptake (VO$_2$) and the oxygen extraction ratio (OER) during daily intermittent machine haemofiltration treatment. Mean values $\pm$ SEM.

patients would have maximally utilised their compensatory mechanisms designed to reduce ICP [14], and thereby be most at risk from developing cerebral oedema. Those patients treated by the continuous modes showed greater stability of ICP than those treated by MHF, and required fewer interventions to control ICP.

Similarly, although the mean arterial blood pressure prior to treatment was less in the continuously treated group, arterial blood pressure was better maintained during the first 5 h of treatment compared to MHF.

A critical cerebral perfusion pressure of 50 mm Hg has been suggested [15], below which cerebral hypoxia develops, while other workers have suggested a value of 60 mm Hg [14] in patients with abnormalities of the blood-brain barrier. In this study the cerebral perfusion pressure was lower in the continuously treated group prior to treatment, but showed greater stability during treatment compared to the MHF group. No patient in the

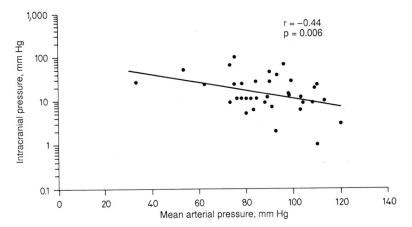

Fig. 5. Relationship between ICP and mean arterial blood pressure (MAP) prior to renal replacement therapy, showing a linear relationship suggesting defective cerebral autoregulation.

continuously treated group, who did not have evidence of increased ICP/ cerebral oedema prior to starting treatment died from cerebral oedema. Whereas in the group treated by MHF 3 of the 6 patients (50%) who subsequently died from cerebral oedema, had a baseline ICP of less than 14 mm Hg and an initial cerebral perfusion pressure greater than 70 mm Hg.

In this group of patients susceptible to developing cerebral oedema, changes in cardiac output and cerebral perfusion pressure can result in cerebral hypoxia and further increases in ICP due to the failure of cerebral autoregulatory mechanisms. In this study the greatest changes in ICP and cerebral perfusion pressure occurred during the first hour of treatment by MHF, at a time when changes in serum osmolality were small. During this period there were marked changes in cardiac output and cerebral oxygen delivery. However, instead of a compensatory increase in the tissue oxygen (cerebral) extraction ratio, tissue oxygen (cerebral) uptake decreased. This would be expected to result in further cerebral hypoxia associated with an increase in ICP secondary to cerebral arteriolar vasodilatation [12]. The small differences observed between CAVHF and CAVHD treatment probably reflected differences in fluid balance and cardiac output during the first hour of treatment. During CAVHD there was no pump (throttle) on the dialysate effluent side to restrict losses, which were typically underestimated during the first hour of treatment.

Previous studies in patients with FHF and acute renal failure using standard haemodialysis treatment reported a high incidence of cerebral oedema/hypoxia [16]. Subsequent studies have shown that even daily intermittent haemofiltration can cause marked increases in ICP [17], which can be reduced by using CAVHF [18]. CAVHF has also been shown superior to intermittent machine treatments in terms of maintaining cerebral perfusion pressure [19], which is of critical importance in patients with cerebral oedema and/or failure of cerebral autoregulation. In these patients the greatest changes in ICP and cerebral perfusion pressure occur within the first hour of treatment [20], and although the fundamental pathophysiology is as yet unknown, these changes are related to a reduction in both cerebral oxygen delivery and uptake, unlike the classical pattern observed in the 'dialysis disequilibrium syndrome' [1]. Although largely controlable, these adverse effects of MHF make it hazardous especially if no ICP monitoring is in place. The continuous modes of treatment are not without their own problems but provide a mode of renal replacement therapy for patients at risk of cerebral oedema which is less hazardous than that offered by intermittent machine-driven haemodialysis/haemofiltration.

Acknowledgements
We wish to thank Prof. M.S. Losowosky for allowing us to report on his patients, and Dr. A.T. Cohen and the nursing staff on the intensive care unit for their support and co-operation during the study. We wish to acknowledge the help and assistance of neurosurgical colleagues, and the continued support of the Yorkshire Kidney Research Fund. A.D. was in receipt of a Yorkshire Kidney Research Fund grant.

References

1   Doyle JE: Extracorporeal Haemodialysis therapy. Springfield, Thomas, 1962.
2   LaGreca G, Dettori P, Biasioli S, Chiaramonte S, Fabris A, Feriani M, Pinna V, Pisani E, Ronco C: Studies on brain density in haemodialysis and peritoneal dialysis. Nephron 1982;31:146–150.
3   Winney RJ, Kean DM, Best JJK, Smith MA: Changes in brain density with haemodialysis. Lancet 1987;ii:1102–1108.
4   Maudsley C: Neurological complications of haemodialysis. Proc R Soc Med 1972;65:871–873.
5   Davenport A, Finn R, Goldsmith HJ: The management of patients with renal failure complicated by cerebral oedema. Blood Purif 1989;7:203–209.
6   Ware AJ, D'Agostino AN, Combes B: Cerebral oedema: A major complication of massive hepatic necrosis. Gastroenterology 1971;61:877–884.
7   Forbes A, Alexander GJM, O'Grady J, Keays R, Gullen R, Dawling S, Williams R: Thiopental infusion in the treatment of intracranial pressure complicating fulminant hepatic failure. Hepatology 1989;3:306–310.
8   Canalese J, Gimson AES, Davis C, Mellon PJ, Davis M, Williams R: Controlled trial of dexamethasone and mannitol for the cerebral oedema of fulminant hepatic failure. Gut 1982;23:625–629.
9   Ede R, Keays R, Williams R: Intracranial pressure monitoring and management of encephalopathy. Care Crit Ill 1989;5:46–48.

10 Wilkinson SP, Weston MJ, Parsons V, Williams R: Dialysis in the treatment of renal failure in patients with liver disease. Clin Nephrol 1977;8:287–292.

11 Sherlock S: Vasodilatation associated with hepatocellular disease: Relation to functional organ failure. Gut 1990;31:365–366.

12 Van Wylen DGL, Park TS, Rubio R, Berne RM: Increases in cerebral interstitial fluid adenosine concentration during hypoxia, local potassium infusion and ischaemia. J Cereb Blood Flow Metab 1986;6:522–528.

13 Davenport A, Will EJ, Davison AM: The effect of posture on intracranial pressure in patients with fulminant hepatic failure and oliguric renal failure following paracetamol (acetaminophen) self-poisoning. Crit Care Med 1990;18:286–289.

14 Price DJ: Intracranial pressure monitoring. Br J Clin Equip 1980;5:92–98.

15 Lassen NA, Christensen MS: Physiology of cerebral blood flow. Br J Anaesthesiol 1976;48:719–734.

16 Silk DBA, Williams R: Experiences in the treatment of fulminant hepatic failure by conservative therapy, charcoal haemoperfusion and polyacrylonitrile membrane haemodialysis. Int J Artif Organs 1978;1:29–33.

17 Davenport A, Will EJ, Davison AM, Cohen AT, Swindells S, Miloszewski KJA, Losowsky MS: Changes in intracranial pressure during machine and continuous haemofiltration in patients with grade IV hepatic encephalopathy. Int J Artif Organs 1989;12:429–434.

18 Davenport A, Will EJ, Swindells S, Losowsky MS: Continuous arteriovenous haemofiltration in patients with hepatic encephalopathy and renal failure. Br Med J 1987;295:1028.

19 Davenport A, Will EJ, Davison AM, Swindells S, Cohen AT, Miloszewski KJA, Losowosky MS: Changes in intracranial pressure during haemofiltration in oliguric patients with grade 4 hepatic encephalopathy. Nephron 1989;53:142–146.

20 Davenport A, Will EJ, Davison AM· Early changes in intracranial pressure during haemofiltration treatment in patients with grade 4 hepatic encephalopathy and acute oliguric renal failure. Nephrol Dial Transplant 1990;5:192–198.

Dr. A. Davenport, Department of Renal Medicine, Southmead Hospital, Westbury on Trym, Bristol BS10 5NP (UK)

Sieberth HG, Mann H, Stummvoll HK (eds): Continuous Hemofiltration.
Contrib Nephrol. Basel, Karger, 1991, vol 93, pp 234–236

Conservative Treatment of Severe Necrotizing Pancreatitis Using Early Continuous Venovenous Hemofiltration

L. Blinzler[a], *J. Haußer*[a], *H. Bödeker*[b], *U. Zaune*[a], *E. Martin*[a],
Ch. Gebhardt[b]

Departments of [a]Anesthesia and [b]General and Thoracic Surgery,
Klinikum Nürnberg, FRG

Severe necrotizing pancreatitis (NP) concerning 10–20% of all acute cases is frequently connected with lethal complications, even when treated surgically. Based on this experience a new therapeutic approach was developed, which aims at conservative treatment in all patients with NP. Cases with proven infection of necrosis, pancreatic abscess or other local complications were excluded.

Patients

Since January 1989 there were 11 patients with a severe clinical course in whom continuous veno-venous hemofiltration (CVVHF) was used. This group only consisted of men aged between 23 and 52 years. The etiological factor of NP was almost always alcoholism.

Routinely performed contrast-enhanced CT scans showed necrosis of the pancreas and the peripancreatic tissue in all patients. Pancreotography also showed pathological findings.

All patients developed multiple organ failure (MOF). Elevated body temperature of more than 39.0 °C, encephalopathy and pulmonary failure were seen in general. Nine patients needed mechanical ventilation. Other organ failures appeared frequently like renal failure, hyperdynamic shock, hepatic failure, thrombopenia and hyperglycemia.

Methods and Materials

This conservative approach consists of three components: critical care basic therapy, prophylactic antibiotics, and the use of CVVHF. The baseline management at the ICU included appropriate oxygen supply, mechanical ventilation, volume replacement, hemodynamic stabilization, parenteral nutrition, gastric suction, prevention of stress ulceration, analgesic drugs, correction of hydroelectrolytic and acid-base disorders, and adequate monitoring.

Primary antibiotic therapy was performed by a cephalosporin of the third generation and metronidazol in combination with selective digestive decontamination.

Patients underwent early hemofiltration, when symptoms of MOF like pulmonary or renal failure occurred.

Vascular access was obtained using a double lumen catheter inserted percutaneously into one of the great veins. CVVHF was done by a roller pump (BSM 22, Hospal) and a

Table 1. Substances possibly eliminated by hemofiltration

	MW Da
C3a	9,000
C5a	11,000
β_2-Microglobulin	11,600
Phospholipase A2	13,600
Interleukin 1	17,000
TNF/cachectin	17,000

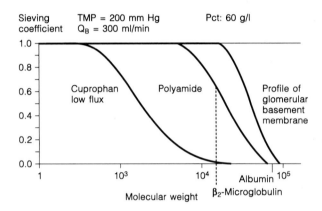

Fig. 1. Sieving coefficient for polyamide measured in plasma.

polyamide hollow fiber membrane filter (FH 66 Hemofilter, Gambro) with blood flow at 200 ml/min. Ultrafiltrate was replaced by isotonic hemofiltration fluid (HF 23, Fresenius) in a postdilution mode. Anticoagulation was achieved by sodium heparin from 0 to 1,500 U/h. Average ultrafiltrate volumes of the patients ranged up from 8,100 to 41,900 ml/day with a mean volume of 23,200 ml/day.

CVVHF was stopped when the symptoms of MOF returned to the normal range. Hemofiltration was performed from 8 to 50 days, on average 14.5 days.

Results

Ten of 11 patients survived. They left ICU after a mean period of 30 days, ranged from 19 to 69 days. One patient died. Results from autopsy showed leukemia, hepatic cirrhosis, severe coronary artery disease and fatal pneumonia.

In spite of septic signs like high temperature and elevated white blood counts there was no evidence of local infection of necrosis. Using CVVHF we saw improvement of pulmonary and renal function within some days. Also initial thrombopenia disappeared.

Discussion

Necrotizing in severe pancreatitis causes an invasion of vasoactive substances and mediators into the systemic circulation. Some of these substances like histamine, serotonin, bradykinin, metabolites of arachidonic acid, phospholipase A_2, anaphylatoxins (C3a, C5a) and cytokines (TNF, IL1) seem to participate in the development of MOF [1, 2, 4, 5].

Therapeutic approaches in NP therefore aim to prevent the genesis of such mediators or to decrease their plasma concentration. The elimination of low-molecular-weight mediators like histamine, serotonin, bradykinin or products of the arachidonic cascade by hemofiltration is probable. The sieving coefficient of the used polyamide membrane allows filtration of higher molecular weight polypeptides (fig. 1, table 1). This is demonstrated for anaphylatoxins [3]. There is evidence that early elimination of TNF prevents septic animals from symptoms of MOF [1]. We presume that lowering of mediator concentrations in the systemic circulation by CVVHF is responsible for the disappearance of MOF in NP.

Whether there is a significant decrease of mediators in the blood by hemofiltrations will be the aim of further investigations.

References

1   Beutler B, Milsark IW, Cerami A: Passive immunization against cachectin/tumor necrosis factor protects mice from lethal effect of endotoxin. Science 1985;229:869–871.
2   Dugernier T, Reynaert MS: Management of severe pancreatitis; in Vincent JL (ed): Update in Intensive Care and Emergency Medicine, Update 1990. Berlin, Springer, 1990, vol 10, pp 698–705.
3   Jorstad S, Smeby LC, Balstad T, Wideroe TE: Generation and removal of anaphylatoxins during hemofiltration with five different membranes. Blood Purif 1988;6:325–335.
4   Rinderknecht H: Fatal pancreatitis, a consequence of excessive leukocyte stimulation? Int J Pancreat 1988;3:105–112.
5   Vollmar B, Waldner H, Schmad J, Conzen P, Habazettl A, Goetz A, Schweiberger L, Brendel W: Arachidonsäuremetabolite bei akuter experimenteller Pankreatitis am Schwein (abstract). Anaesthesist 1989;38(Suppl):310.

Dr. L. Blinzler, Institut für Anästhesiologie, Klinikum Nürnberg, Flurstrasse 17, D–W–8500 Nürnberg 91 (FRG)

Sieberth HG, Mann H, Stummvoll HK (eds): Continuous Hemofiltration.
Contrib Nephrol. Basel, Karger, 1991, vol 93, pp 237–240

Isolation of Low-Molecular-Weight Peptides in Hemofiltrated Patients with Cardiogenic Shock: A New Aspect of Myocardial Depressant Substances

F. Coraim, W. Trubel, R. Ebermann, T. Werner

Department of Anesthesiology and Intensive Care, University of Vienna, Austria

The existence of negative inotropic substances in the circulating blood of various shock states in humans and animals are confirmed. In the bioassay using an isolated heart preparation all these factors have been shown to exert a negative inotropic activity. At present, the physiological properties of these factors seem to be well characterized [1], whereas their chemical structures have not been elucidated so far. In our previous studies [2], we have investigated the inotropic activity of proteogenetic amino acids. Their molecular weight, as far as it is described, varies between 250 and a few thousand daltons [1]. Consequently, therefore, we investigated other low molecular weight peptides with a different chemical structure, consisting mainly of acidic amino acids and/or cysteine in respect to their negative inotropic activity. The occurrence of such low-molecular-weight peptides built into larger peptides or proteins is discussed and finally we put forward a hypothesis under which conditions these small peptides may develop a physiological relevance in cardiopathology.

Material and Methods

The negative inotropic response of an isolated guinea pig papillary muscle in respect to asparic acid, glutamic acid and cysteine was investigated. Synthetic peptides (Sigma, Munich, FRG) with a similar molecular weight and well-known chemical structure (dipeptides formed by combination of the amino acids asparic acid and glutamic acid; all listed in table 2) were compared in negative inotropic effects to plasma samples and the corresponding hemofiltrates of 9 cardiogenic shock patients and 3 control plasma samples. All probes were assayed in 1:1 dilution with Krebs-Henseleit (KH) solution for negative inotropic activity according to a modification of the method of Lefer [1], already used in our previous study [2]. The fractions of the chromatographic separations were lyophilized and reconstitued with KH solution before the bioassay. In the bioassay using isolated guinea pig papillary muscle, the MDF-

Table 1. Reduction of inotropic activity (%) by human shock samples

Sample No.	Shock plasma %	Hemofiltrates %	Control plasma %
1	30.5	30.4	0.1
2	31.3	31.0	0.0
3	29.5	29.6	0.1
4	35.4	35.6	
5	29.1	29.3	
6	38.5	39.0	
7	25.0	25.0	
8	20.0	21.1	
9	26.1	26.0	
	x = 29.5 ± 5.4 Vx = 18.66	x = 29.7 ± 5.5 Vx = 18.21	

Table 2. Selected amino acids (all L configuration) and peptides with a negative inotropic effect in the bioassay (%) and their borderline concentrations (= concentration leading to an alteration of the initial contractile forces of at least 10%)

Asparic acid	18 ± 1.8	500 *mM*
Glutamic acid	17.5 ± 0.8	500 *µM*
Asparagine	17.3 ± 1.2	10 *µM*
Glutamine	17.3 ± 1.3	10 *µM*
Cysteine	17.4 ± 2.0	500 *µM*
Asp-Glu	17.3 ± 0.8	500 *µM*
Glu-Glu	17.5 ± 0.8	500 *µM*
Asp-Asp	18 ± 0.5	500 *µM*
Glu-Ala-Glu	16.4 ± 1.4	800 *µM*
Glutathione (oxidative form)	13.8 ± 1.6	1 mM
Glutathione (reductive form)	13.8 ± 1.4	1 mM
Glu-Ala-Glu-Asn	19 ± 1.5	2 mM
Val-Glu-Asp-Glu	22.4 ± 0.8	1 mM
Val-Glu-Glu-Ala-Glu	22 ± 1.4	900 *µM*
Lys-Glu-Glu-Ala-Glu	13.8 ± 0.9	2 mM
Cardiotoxine	22.8 ± 0.9	10 *µM*

activity was recorded as percent inhibition in developed tension of the papillary muscle at double-concentrated KH solution to come to the borderline concentration for a negative inotropy. Negative inotropic activity of each substance was quoted when the alteration of the initial contractile force was at least 10%. Statistical evaluation was performed by use of the student's t-test.

Results

The numerical results of this comparative study are listed in tables 1 and 2. Compared to the control plasma all investigated substances initiated a significant decline of active tension (AT) below the corresponding values of the untreated muscles ($p < 0.01$; Student's t test). The negative inotropic activity of these peptides was similar to that of the free constituents the peptides were composed of (table 2).

Discussion

In this study the effect of some small peptides on the mechanical performance of isolated guinea pig papillary muscles was demonstrated. The negative inotropic activity of the acid amino acids (Glu and Asp) we found recently furnished the incentive to investigate the inotropic activity of peptides consisting mainly of acid amino acids. In a series of experiments we tested the effect of the dipeptides formed by the combination of Asp and Glu: Asp-Asp, Glu-Glu, and Asp-Glu. As expected, no difference was found in respect to inotropic activity in comparison to the activity of their constituents (table 2). Introduction of a hydrophobic amino acid results in a decrease of active tension (AT) of guinea pig papillary muscle. The tetrapeptide Val-Glu-Asp-Glu decreased the AT at a concentration of 1 mM. This means that it is twice as effective as the tetrapeptide Glu-Ala-Glu-Asn tested before. The pentapeptide Val-Glu-Glu-Asp-Glu showed to be as similarly effective as the tetrapeptide Val-Glu-Asp-Glu (table 2). Valine as the apolar constitutent of those peptides might be replaceable by leucine and isoleucine. One of the main reasons for the necessity of the presence of apolar amino acids in a negative inotropic-acting peptide is its diminished diffusion rate in the predominant aqueous system. Another one might be that the binding with the target tissue is facilitated and the acidic environment mediated by the amino acids constitutents can be localized at a certain point.

Physiological Relevance. All the peptides tested in the bioassay occur in polypeptides of known structure. The sequences Glu-Ala-Glu, Val-Glu-Glu-Ala-Glu, Glu-Ala-Glu-Asp are all found on the C-terminal end of thymosin [3].

Although PTH is a predominantly basic polypeptide in respect to its amino acid composition there is at the C-terminus of this peptide a region which consists mainly of amino acids [4, 5].

Another prominent peptide with obvious accumulation of a polar and acidic amino acids is the C chain of human proinsulin. The C peptide serves in most cases as a very useful indicator for insulin release and has a much longer lifetime than insulin itself [6]. Interestingly, the human C peptide has an amino acid sequence very similar to that found in the PTH molecule. Under the clinical conditions of multiple forms of shock unphysiological high levels of amino acids and small peptides are produced [7]. The circulatory shock for example is characterized by a variety of alterations of intra- and extracellular fluid metabolism. There is a marked increase in peptides and free amino acid concentration. The formation of these metabolites is closely associated with the activation of lysosomal enzymes. The total plasma proteolysis and the amino N activity is correlated very closely. The present study furnishes a physiological model by which negative inotropy and peptide structure can be correlated.

References

1   Lefer AM: Properties of Cardioinhibitory factors produced in shock, Fed Proc 1978;37:2734.
2   Coraim F, Pauser G, Stellwag F: Positive Beeinflussung der Hämodynamik bei postkardiochirurgischen Patienten durch die Hämofiltration. Eine verbesserte Methodik zur Darstellung des Myocardial Depressant Factor (MDF) im Hämofiltrat. Anaesthesist 1985;34:236.
3   Greene LJ, Shapanka R, Glenn TM, et al: Isolation of Myocardial Depressant Factor from Plasma of Dogs in Hemorrhagic Shock. Biochim Biophys Acta 1977;491:275.
4   Hashimoto K, Nakagawa Y, Shibuya T, et al: Effects of Parathyroid Hormone and related polypeptides on the heart and coronary circulation of dogs. J Cardiovasc Pharmacol 1981;2:668.
5   Potts JT, Kronenberg HM, Rosenblatt M: Parathyroid Hormone: Chemistry, Biosynthesis and Mode of Action. Adv Prot Chem 1982;35:23.
6   Rohdes CJ, Halban PA: The Intracellular handling of Insulin-related peptides in isolated pancreatic islets. Biochem J 1988;251:23.
7   Leffler IN, Litvin Y, Barenholz Y, et al: Proteolysis in formation of a myocardial depressant factor during shock. Am J Physiol 1973;224:824.

F.I. Coraim, MD, Lustkandlgasse 18/5, A–1090 Vienna (Austria)

Sieberth HG, Mann H, Stummvoll HK (eds): Continuous Hemofiltration.
Contrib Nephrol. Basel, Karger, 1991, vol 93, pp 241–244

Extracorporeal Treatment of Ascitic Fluid and Intraperitoneal Reinfusion in Patients with Refractory Ascites

A. Brendolan[a], *C. Ronco*[a], *M. Feriani*[a], *S. Chiaramonte*[a],
L. Bragantini[a], *M. Dal Santo*[b], *L. Lora*[b], *A. D'Alessandro*[b],
G. La Greca[a]

Departments of [a]Nephrology and [b]Medicine 3, St. Bortolo Hospital, Vicenza, Italy

The invasive methods utilized to reduce ascitic fluid and its rate of production are the external drainage by paracentesis [1], the peritoneovenous shunts (LeVeen) [2] or the pumped evacuation of peritoneal fluid and reinfusion in a peripheral vein after concentration [3]. These techniques may present several drawbacks: loss of plasma proteins and further worsening of renal failure, increased risk of cardiovascular overload and coagulative disturbances [4].

The aim of this study is to present a simple technique for extracorporeal concentration and reinfusion of ascitic fluid in the peritoneal cavity.

Methods and Patients

Methods. We have utilized a special equipment CURA (Amicon, Danvers, Mass., USA), as shown in figure 1, utilizing only gravity as a driving force.

After institution of a reliable peritoneal access, the CURA machine operates without pumps, utilizing a unit consisting of a polysulfone hemofilter (0.6 m^2) and a closed circuit connected to the peritoneal access. Ascitic fluid is drained by gravity from the peritoneum through the filter to a bag used as a transit reservoir. When the transit bag is full, the unit consisting of ultrafilter, transit bag and special tubing set is automatically raised to a height sufficient to let the fluid flowing back to the abdominal cavity. Mainly during this step a remarkable ultrafiltration takes place through the filter. Ultrafiltration is enhanced by the negative pressure created in the filtrate compartment by the difference in height between the filter and the drainage bag placed at the bottom of the machine. The proteins in the ascitic fluid are retained and returned to the patient. The machine repeats automatically the cycle as many times as necessary.

Population. Seventeen patients with refractory ascites, 13 with alcoholic cirrhosis, 4 with hepatocellular carcinoma were treated utilizing the above-described machine. All patients had a body fluid overload with an overweight ranging from 8 to 15 kg (the fluid overload was calculated according to the formula: plasma Na/140 × 60% body weight). Blood, urine and

Table 1. Chemical parameters

Patient	Number of treatments	Cycles/treatment	Total ultra-filtrate	Plasma Na mEg/l		Total plasma protein, g/l		Ascitic fluid total protein		Urine Na mEg/l		Urine volume ml/24 h		Therapeutic response
				pre	post	pre	post	pre	post	pre	post	pre	post	
M.L.	5	15	3,930	131	139	4.5	6.1	1.6	3.4	40	49	1,500	3,000	+ +
M.L.	1	16	1,750	134	136	5.8	7.1	0.8	5.0	39	65	800	2,000	+ + +
Z.L.	1	14	1,350	139	137	7.0	7.2	0.6	2.1	36	54	1,900	2,700	+ + +
R.S.	2	13	3,350	122	124	7.5	7.6	2.4	4.6	26	176	600	2,000	+ +
B.V.	3	22	8,220	129	130	6.6	6.8	0.7	1.0	80	109	800	1,600	+ +
R.P.	1	25	1,120	129	130	6.6	6.6	2.5	6.1	85	132	900	1,650	+
F.Z.	1	10	500	118	122	5.7	6.0	3.1	6.6	55	87	700	1,200	+
R.S.	3	9	2,600	122	123	7.3	7.7	1.3	1.8	35	63	1,500	2,000	+
A.C.	2	15	3,000	128	130	6.7	7.1	1.8	3.5	48	90	800	1,500	+
O.G.	3	15	6,500	127	129	5.7	6.3	3.7	4.3	56	92	600	1,700	+
F.I.	1	12	1,300	129	130	5.2	5.7	2.4	3.8	62	88	500	1,200	+ −
B.G.	1	12	1,350	128	128	5.6	6.1	2.6	4.2	38	65	600	1,200	+ −
F.A.	1	14	1,430	132	134	5.6	5.8	1.2	2.6	25	64	400	1,100	+ +
R.A.	3	20	4,500	131	131	5.9	6.0	2.7	3.5	39	55	500	850	+ −
P.C.	3	18	5,600	127	129	5.4	6.2	1.4	2.7	29	95	700	2,000	+ +
T.A.	1	14	1,300	129	130	5.7	6.3	1.2	2.5	33	80	950	1,700	+ +
V.C.	1	16	700	129	129	5.4	5.5	2.6	3.1	48	62	600	950	+ −
Mean		15.2	2,858	128.3	130.1	6.0	6.5	1.9	3.5	45.2	84.4	844.1	1,667.6	
SD		±4.1	±2,227	±4.7	±4.6	±0.8	±0.6	±0.9	±1.6	±12.2	±22.2	±411.5	±585.2	
Significance				$p < 0.01$		$p < 0.001$		$p < 0.001$		$p < 0.001$		$p < 0.001$		

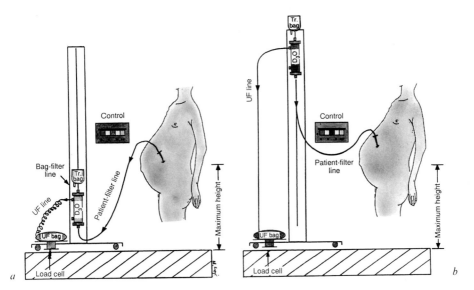

Fig. 1. *a* First step of the cycle: the filter is placed in a lower position and fluid withdrawal from the peritoneal cavity takes place. The transit (Tr.) bag is progressively filled. *b* Second step of the cycle: the filter is raised with the transit bag above the patient and the fluid is returned to the peritoneal cavity after concentration due to ultrafiltration (UF).

ascitic fluid samples were taken at the beginning and at the end of each session to measure electrolytes and total protein. We performed a total of 33 extracorporeal treatments.

Results

The operational and chemical parameters obtained in our patients are listed in table 1. No significant variations in blood pressure and in the other biochemical parameters measured were registered and all patients tolerated the treatment without clinical or technical complications. 41% of patients had satisfactory clinical results with reduction of ascites after one session. They could be easily managed with diuretics and inotropic drugs without critical relapses up to 6 months from the procedure. In 29% body fluid control and the reduction of ascites formation could be achieved after 2 or more sessions of treatment. 30% of patients showed poor results. Most of them had liver cancer.

Discussion

Ultrafiltration of ascitic fluid and reinfusion of the concentrate in the abdominal cavity seem to offer several advantages in comparison with other techniques commonly used in the treatment of refractory ascites. This treatment reduces the remarkable protein loss linked to the extraction of ascitic fluid. Despite a high protein concentration in the fluid reinfused into the peritoneal cavity, the rate of ascites formation is unexpectedly reduced. A possible increase in lymphatic reabsorption might allow the passage of proteins from the peritoneal cavity into the venous bloodstream. This hypothesis could explain, at least in part, the reduction in the rate of ascitic fluid production and the increased clinical response to medications after the extracorporeal procedure.

In conclusion, the technique seems to be safe, clinically well tolerated and efficient for the treatment of patients with ascites refractory to other therapies.

References

1   Quintero E, Gines P, Arroyo V, et al: Paracentesis versus diuretics in the treatment of cirrhosis with tense ascites. Lancet 1985;i:611–612.
2   Epstein M: Role of the peritoneovenous shunt in the management of ascites and the hepato-renal syndrome; in Epstein M (ed): The Kidney in Liver Disease. New York, Elsevier, 1983, pp 538–600.
3   Inoue I, Yamazaki Z, Oda T, Sugiura M, Wada T. Fujika Y, Hayano F: Treatment of intractable ascites by continous reinfusion of the sterilized cell-free and concentrated ascitic fluid. Trans ASAIO 1977;23:699–702.
4   Landini S, Coli U, Fracasso A, Morachiello P, Righetto F, Scanferla F, Gallenda F, Bazzato G: Spontaneous ascites filtration and reinfusion (SAFR) as ambulatory chronic treatment of hepato-renal syndrome. Trans ASAIO 1985;31:439–443.

Dr. A. Brendolan, Department of Nephrology, St. Bortolo Hospital, I–36100 Vicenza (Italy)

Sieberth HG, Mann H, Stummvoll HK (eds): Continuous Hemofiltration.
Contrib Nephrol. Basel, Karger, 1991, vol 93, pp 245–249

Continuous Renal Replacement in Infants and Toddlers

Randall D. Jenkins[a], *Harold L. Harrison*[a], *Elizabeth C. Jackson*[b], *James E. Funk*[c]

[a]Department of Pediatrics, University of Louisville, Ky.; Departments of [b]Pediatrics and [c]Mechanical Engineering, University of Kentucky, Ky., USA

In pediatric patients, continuous renal replacement therapy (CRRT) such as continuous arteriovenous hemofiltration (CAVH) or continuous arteriovenous hemodialysis (CAVHD) have been reported to be relatively trouble free [1]. We have found that these procedures present technical problems as well as some operational characteristics not previously reported. The purpose of this report is to elucidate some of these technical problems and differences which occur with CRRT in small pediatric patients.

Methods

A retrospective review was conducted of 12 patients under 4 years of age who were treated with CAVH or CAVHD, and in whom adequate data were available. CAVH was performed with the method of Lauer et al. [2]. CAVHD was performed in a manner similar to that of Sigler and Teehan [3]. Dialysate for CAVHD was either lactate, acetate, or bicarbonate based. Heparin was given by hourly bolus of 10–20 U/kg and was adjusted to keep activated clotting time greater than 170 s. Dialysate inflow, outflow, and ultrafiltrate were controlled by intravenous infusion pump. Dialysate inflows were varied between 1 and 6 ml/min.

Bloodflow was calculated by the method of Lauer et al. [2]. Urea clearance in CAVH systems was considered to be the same as UFR since the sieving coefficient for urea is 1.05 [4]. In CAVHD systems, urea clearance was calculated according to the dialysate side method of Schneider and Geronemus [4]. Catheter inner diameter was determined by a previously published method [5]. The CAVH systems which were used are shown in table 1.

Vascular access was obtained using four different types of catheter. A polyvinyl chloride (PVC) thick-wall, 5-Fr umbilical vessel infusion catheter was used initially for umbilical vascular access in 2 patients. Polyurethane 16-gauge, 16-cm catheters (ID 0.95 mm) were placed in either the femoral or the umbilical vessels in 4 patients. In another patient, 4-Fr introducer sheaths (ID 1.6 mm) were used. Thin-wall, 7.5-cm, 5.5-Fr polyurethane catheters (ID 1.45 mm) were placed in 6 patients.

Table 1. Results of CRRT in 12 infants and toddlers

Age group	Patient No.	Modality	System	Access route	Access type	Q_b ml/min	Cl_{urea} ml/min	Comment
NB	1	CAVH	Amicon D20	umbilical	PVC	3	0.3	frequent stasis
NB	2	CAVH	Amicon D20	umbilical	PVC	3	0.4	frequent stasis
NB	3	Both	Amicon Mini	umbilical/femoral	PU	4	0.2	frequent stasis
NB	4	Both	Amicon Mini	femoral	PU	3	0.6*	high K^+ on CAVH
NB	5	CAVHD	Amicon Mini	umbilical	PU	18	0.7	edema formation
NB	6	CAVHD	Gambro FH22	umbilical	PU	+	2.4	no problems
INF	7	CAVHD	Gambro FH22	femoral	SHEATH	41	2.9	kinking of sheath
INF	8	CAVHD	Amicon Mini	femoral	PUTW	25	0.8	no problems
INF	9	CAVHD	Amicon Mini	femoral	PUTW	30	1.4	no problems
INF	10	CAVHD	Gambro FH22	femoral	PUTW	++	3.2	no problems
TOD	11	CAVHD	Amicon D20	femoral	PUTW	8	1.6	poor flow
TOD	12	CAVHD	Amicon Mini Plus	femoral	PUTW	30	2.9	no problems

NB = Newborn; INF = infant; TOD = toddler; *0.2 for CAVH; + = estimated to be 5–10 ml/min; ++ = estimated to be 20–30 ml/min; PVC = polyvinyl chloride 5-Fr umbilical catheter (ID 0.7–0.9 mm); PU = polyurethane 16-gauge, 16-cm catheter (ID 0.95 mm); SHEATH = 4-Fr introducer sheath (ID 1.6 mm); PUTW = polyurethane thin-wall CAVH catheter (ID 1.45 mm).

Results

System bloodflow for patients 1 and 2 was very low (table 1). Both patients had umbilical PVC catheters for vascular access. Both systems suffered from recurrent flow stasis as manifested by very slow arterial bloodflow and elevated postfilter hematocrit (as high as 95) and separation of plasma from red cells. When the 16-gauge catheters were used, (patients 3–6) bloodflow was higher (3–18 ml/min), resulting in a decreased tendency for flow stasis and clotting. When introducer sheaths were used in one infant, bloodflow was excellent (41 ml/min) soon after placement; however, these devices twisted and bent easily, usually resulting in permanent obstruction and need for replacement. In the remaining 5 patients, the thin-wall, 5.5-Fr catheters were used with good bloodflow and no recurrent flow stasis (table 1).

Urea clearance was low as was bloodflow in all 4 patients treated with CAVH, as shown in table 1. Patient 4 developed symptomatic hyperkalemia while being treated with CAVH. This problem was corrected promptly by changing from CAVH to CAVHD, increasing potassium clearance from 0.2 to 0.6 ml/min. Urea clearance in the four CAVHD Minifilter® systems varied between 0.6 and 1.4 ml/min and appeared to be related to bloodflow rate. Urea clearance was substantially higher for both the Minifilter Plus® and FH-22® systems as compared to the Minifilter systems (table 1).

Mechanical problems other than recurrent flow stasis included multiple disconnections of the ultrafiltrate port adaptor of the FH-22 hemofilter. Also, the intravenous infusion pumps alarmed frequently, both for appropriate and inappropriate reasons. In 1 patient, bypass of the alarm system resulted in delivery of dialysate across the membrane to the patient when the 'out' pump was inoperative. In patient 5, the actual weight loss of the patient was less than one would have anticipated given the dialysate pump settings. Frequent alarms of the 'out' pump were thought to cause the fluid imbalance. Two episodes of bleeding related to anticoagulation occurred; however, neither episode resulted in discontinuation of therapy.

Discussion

A major difference in operation of these small pediatric CRRT systems compared to adult systems is the relatively high catheter flow resistance in pediatric systems and consequent dependence of system bloodflow on catheter flow resistance [5]. Although unreported until now, the problem of repeated flow stasis requiring frequent hemofilter changes has been seen by others in pediatric CRRT applications [personal commun, Steven Alexander, Dallas; Michael Leone, Portland; Bryson Waldo, Birmingham]. These data also indicate that this problem may be avoided with use of catheters of low flow resistance. A preliminary report suggests that the problem of repeated flow stasis is due to a positive feedback between UFR, venous blood viscosity, and transmembrane pressure in some situations when postfilter hematocrit becomes elevated [6]. This problem is much more likely to occur with high flow resistance catheters.

Catheters should not be chosen simply on the basis of reported gauge or French size. Pediatric catheters, particularly umbilical catheters, of supposed same size were shown to have as much as 37% variability of ID [5]. For these reasons, standard thick-wall umbilical catheters are not desirable for use in CRRT systems. The 16-gauge catheters which we used are only marginally acceptable in providing adequate bloodflow. The 5.5-Fr thin-wall CAVH catheters were preferred because they provided substantially higher bloodflows without the problem of repeated flow stasis or mechanical obstruction. Ronco et al. [7] have reported that short (2–3 mm) catheters of 18–20 gauge give acceptable bloodflow results for CAVH in the newborn.

Urea clearance and UFR in the CAVH systems was not related to bloodflow. This was also the finding of Ronco et al [7]. In adult CAVHD systems, urea clearance is approximated by dialysate flow rate [3]. This is not so in our pediatric systems because bloodflow is not much higher than dialysate flow, and hemofilters used have small membrane surface areas. The relationships which govern CAVHD clearance in pediatric systems have not been worked out yet.

Because our patient groups were small and not comparable, a general comparison of CAVH and CAVHD was not made. However, for the Minifilter system, urea clearance with CAVHD was higher than could be obtained with CAVH. Others have also reported increased solute clearance with CAVHD as compared to CAVH in pediatric patients [8].

References

1 Zobel G, Ring E, Zobel V: Continuous arteriovenous renal replacement systems for critically ill children. Pediatr Nephrol 1989;3:140–143.

2 Lauer A, Saccaggi A, Ronco C, Belledonne M, Glabman S, Bosch JP: Continuous arteriovenous hemofiltration in the critically ill patient. Ann Intern Med 1983;99:455–460.

3 Sigler MH, Teehan BP: Solute transport in continuous hemodialysis: A new treatment for acute renal failure. Kidney Int 1987;32:562–571.

4 Schneider NS, Geronemus RP: Continuous arteriovenous hemodialysis. Kidney Int 1988;33:S-159–S-162.

5 Jenkins RD, Kuhn RJ, Funk JE: Clinical implications of catheter variability in neonatal continuous arteriovenous hemofiltration. ASAIO Trans 1988;11:108–111.

6 Jenkins RD, Funk JE, Kuhn RJ: Etiology of poor performance in pediatric CAVH systems. Book of Abstracts, VIII Congr Int Pediatric Nephrology Assoc, Toronto, August 1989; p 18.016.

7   Ronco C, Brendolan A, Bragantini L, Chiaramonte S, Feriani M, Fabris A, Dell'Aquila
     R, La Greca G: Treatment of acute renal failure in newborns by continuous arterio-
     venous hemofiltration. Kidney Int 1986;29:908–915.
8   Assadi FK: Treatment of acute renal failure in an infant by continuous arteriovenous
     hemodialysis. Pediatr Nephrol 1988;2:320–322.

Dr. Randall Jenkins, Department of Pediatrics, School of Medicine,
University of Louisville, Louisville, KY 40292 (USA)

Sieberth HG, Mann H, Stummvoll HK (eds): Continuous Hemofiltration.
Contrib Nephrol. Basel, Karger, 1991, vol 93, pp 250–253

Parenteral Nutrition during Continuous Arteriovenous Hemofiltration in Critically Ill Anuric Children

M. Kuttnig, G. Zobel, E. Ring, M. Trop

Department of Pediatrics, University of Graz, Austria

Critically ill children with acute renal failure (ARF) are often severely catabolic [1]. If anuria persists, or is associated with other organ system failures, body protein depletion results, which may progress to protein and caloric malnutrition. This is associated with reduced total body protein synthesis, negative protein-N balance, and increased utilization of amino acids (AA). This phenomenon might be a major contributing factor to the high mortality in ARF [2]. Adequate nutritional support is limited because of the body's poor tolerance to large fluid volumes [3]. Continuous arteriovenous hemofiltration (CAVH) allows full parenteral nutrition, without the risk of fluid overload or worsening uremic toxicity. The aim of this report is to show urea nitrogen appearance (UNA), protein nitrogen balance (protein-N balance) and AA balance in 11 critically ill anuric children during total parenteral nutrition (TPN) and CAVH.

Methods

All patients received TPN with glucose, essential AA and non-essential AA (EAA, ENAA), in 7 patients intravenous fat solution was given. All infants and children received commercial AA solutions with a ratio of EAA to ENAA of 1:1.05 and 1:1.53, respectively (Aminomel Baby[R], Aminomel optimal pur[R], Leopold Corp., Graz, Austria). Electrolytes, minerals and vitamins were added according to standard guidelines. For CAVH different filter systems of Polysulfone (Amicon Corp., Lexington, Mass., USA) and Polyamide (Gambro Corp., Hechingen, FRG) were used. Extracorporeal blood volume varied from 9 to 60 ml. Usually, heparin and/or prostacycline was infused. Ultrafiltrate (UF) was collected in a calibrated bag, measured every hour. UF chemistry was analyzed from a portion of the 24-hour UF.

Analytical Procedures: Calculations. Serum urea nitrogen and creatinine were analyzed twice a day from blood samples and UF. Ultrafiltrate urea nitrogen (UNN) excretion was accepted as representative of total nitrogen loss. AA were determined on a daily basis in serum and UF, using an AA analyzer (Biotronic Corp., Frankfurt, FRG). No attempt was made to determine or correct the nitrogen losses through stool, skin, etc. UNA was calculated as the sum of urea nitrogen in UF and change in body urea nitrogen. The estimate of the urea compartment was usually taken as 60% of body weight. Protein-N balance was calculated as nitrogen intake minus UNA. Data are given as mean ± SEM. No statistical comparisons were made because of the small number of patients.

Results

The clinical data of the patients are described in table 1. Nitrogen intake ranged from 0.11 ± 0.04 on day 1 to 0.26 ± 0.07 g/kg/day on day 7, nonprotein calories from 28.4 ± 11.3 on day 1 to 66.4 ± 9.6 kcal/kg/day on day 7. During CAVH mean creatinine and serum urea nitrogen decreased from 3.61 ± 0.94 to 2.42 ± 0.45 mg/dl and from 77.16 ± 15 to 54.86 ± 6.36 mg/dl, respectively. Mean UNA was 183.09 ± 32.2 mg/kg/day. After 7 days of CAVH and TPN, 9 patients had a positive cumulative protein-N balance of 287 ± 68.5 mg/kg and 2 a negative balance of 942.5 ± 113.1 mg/kg. Mean protein-N balance was positive from day 3 on, as shown in figure 1. Mean AA loss in the UF was 0.159 ± 0.0089 g/kg/day, which is 13.6 ± 1.47% of infused AA. Mean ultrafiltrate/serum ratio of AA was 0.9 ± 0.0043. No significant changes in serum AA were noted. Four patients, 3 with a positive, 1 with a negative nitrogen balance, died without recovery of renal function, because of progressive multiple organ system failure (MOSF).

Discussion

As enteral nutrition is often not feasible in critically ill children and TPN must be restricted to avoid fluid overload, adequate nutrition is impossible and results in rapid nutritional depletion. The nutritional goal is to maintain organ status and promote renal function recovery without aggravating the metabolic disturbances. As the actual requirements for nitrogen and energy intake are unknown in patients with ARF, UNA can be used as an indicator for adequate nitrogen and energy intake [4]. In adults, UNA exceeding 5 g/day (70 mg/kg/day of a 70-kg patient) is indicative for hypermetabolism [5]. In 1982, Mickell [6] reported a mean urea nitrogen excretion of 171 ± 89 (mean ± 2 SD) mg/kg/day in critically ill children. In our patients with ARF or MOSF and CAVH, mean UNA and UUN exceeded 180 mg/kg/day. CAVH is a continuous extracorporeal replacement technique based on convective transport that maintains normal composition of the extracorporeal fluid and allows high volume and energy intake. In normal subjects, the loss of free AA via urine is about 2–3% of the supply [3]. Studies on AA balance in adults with CAVH report a loss of free AA via UF about 2–5% of the daily supply [3, 7]. In our patients, the loss of free AA via UF was markedly higher than that reported in adults. Finally, CAVH allows abnormal plasma AA concentra-

Table 1. Clinical and operational data of 11 patients during TPN and CAVH (mean ± 2 SD)

Patient No.	Sex	Age years	BW kg	Cause of ARF
1	m	0.03	3.5	ischemic
2	m	0.12	3.5	ischemic
3	m	1.5	10	ischemic
4	m	1.4	11.0	sepsis
5	m	3	15.0	sepsis
6	m	10	43	hemolytic uremic syndrome
7	f	11	59	glomerulonephritis
8	m	12	40	rhabdomyolysis
9	f	16	66	hepatorenal syndrome
10	m	1.2	10	nephrosis, sepsis
11	m	6.0	20	ischemic

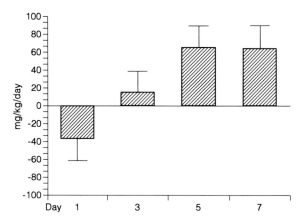

Fig. 1. Protein-N balance under TPN and CAVH (n = 11, mean ± SEM).

tions to be restored, as elimination of AA with high plasma concentrations is much higher than with low plasma concentrations. Because of this fine balancing system, no significant imbalances of plasma AA were observed in our patients. In 1986, Bartlett [8] reported the beneficial effect of a positive energy balance in 29 surgical patients with ARF and CAVH. In contrast to this study, we could not find any correlation between a positive cumulative protein-N balance and recovery of renal function and final outcome in patients with ARF or MOSF. In our patients, outcome was directly correlated to a persisting or progressing MOSF. In conclusion, CAVH

Additional organ system failure	Duration of CAVH h	Ultrafiltration rate ml/min/m^2	Recovery of renal function/ survival
2	160	6.39 ± 1.9	no/no
4	432	4.73 ± 2.1	yes/yes
2	288	4.10 ± 2.9	yes/yes
4	216	14.90 ± 3.7	yes/yes
4	216	4.00 ± 0.81	no/no
3	274	8.60 ± 2.46	yes/yes
0	288	6.34 ± 2.12	yes/yes
3	432	5.50 ± 0.95	yes/yes
5	312	9.60 ± 1.52	no/no
2	176	13.60 ± 2.7	yes/yes
3	456	10.4 ± 2.1	no/no

allows full nutritional support in children with ARF or MOSF without worsening azotemia and fluid balance. It will balance the serum AA. A positive nitrogen balance seems to have no benefit on recovery of renal function. The final outcome depends on the underlying disease.

References

1 Feinstein EI, Blumenkrantz MJ, Healy M, Koffler A, Silberman M, Massry SG, Kopple JD: Clinical and metabolic responses to parenteral nutrition in acute renal failure. Medicine 1981;60:124.

2 Mault JR, Dekert RE, Bartlett RH: Starvation: A major contributor to mortality in acute renal failure? Trans Am Artif Intern Organs 1983;29:390.

3 Schmitz JE, Seeling W, Altemeyer KH, Grünert A, Ahnefeld FW: The parenteral nutrition of hypercatabolic patients during continuous arteriovenous hemofiltration (CAVH); in Sieberth HG, Mann H (eds): Continuous Arteriovenous Hemofiltration (CAVH). Int Conf CAVH, Aachen, 1984, Basel, Karger, 1985, p 204.

4 Takala J: Nutrition in acute renal failure. Crit Care Clin 1987;3:155.

5 Kopple JD, Cianciaruso B: The role of nutrition in acute renal failure (ARF); in Andreucci (ed): Acute Renal Failure (ARF): Pathophysiology, Prevention and Treatment. The Hague, Nijhoff, 1984, chap 22.

6 Mickel JJ: Urea nitrogen excretion in critically ill children. Pediatrics 1982;70:949.

7 Druml W: Amino acid metabolism and amino acid supply in acute renal failure; in Sieberth HG, Mann H (eds): Continuous Arteriovenous Hemofiltration (CAVH). Int Conf CAVH, Aachen, 1984. Basel, Karger, 1985, p 231.

8 Bartlett R: Nutrition in acute renal failure: Treatment made possible by CAVH; in Paganini EP (ed): Acute Continuous Renal Replacement Therapy. Boston, Martinus Nijhoff, 1986, p 173.

Dr. Martin Kuttnig, Department of Pediatrics, University of Graz, Auenbruggerplatz 30, A–8036 Graz (Austria)

Sieberth HG, Mann H, Stummvoll HK (eds): Continuous Hemofiltration.
Contrib Nephrol. Basel, Karger, 1991, vol 93, pp 254–256

High-Performance Continuous Arteriovenous Hemofiltration in Infants with the New Minifilter Plus

C. Ronco, A. Brendolan, L. Bragantini, C. Crepaldi, R. Dell'Aquila,
M. Milan, M. Feriani, S. Chiaramonte, P. Conz, G. La Greca

Department of Nephrology, St. Bortolo Hospital, Vicenza, Italy

The main goal of a Minifilter design for continuous arteriovenous hemofiltration/hemodialysis (CAVH/CAVHD) in infants is to maintain a low priming volume together with a low hydraulic resistance to spontaneous circulation. In the last years a new Minifilter has been created being especially oriented for CAVH treatment in infants [1]. Recently, a further improvement in performance has been achieved with the new Minifilter plus. Both Minifilter standard and Minifilter plus consist of hollow fibers with a large inner diameter.

The hydraulic characteristics of the two filters and their clinical performances are reported here in a series of in vitro and in vivo studies.

Materials and Methods

The fibers of the Minifilter standard and Minifilter plus have inner diameters of 1,000 and 570 μm, respectively. The surface areas of the Minifilter standard and Minifilter plus are 150 and 800 cm^2, respectively; the priming volumes are 6 and 15 ml.

The in vitro studies were carried out with the sequence and circuit previously described [2]. The in vivo studies have been performed in 16 infants with acute renal failure treated with CAVH/CAVHD. CAVH was performed according to the standard technique [3]. CAVHD was done using a dialysate flow ranging from 3 to 10 ml/min.

Results

The hydraulic properties of the two filters are summarized in figure 1. The Minifilter plus maintains a remarkably low resistance. Therefore, the blood flow recorded at a given perfusion pressure is similar to that obtained at the same pressure in the Minifilter standard. The pressure profile inside the two filters at different blood flows is similar. In fact, the Minifilter plus maintains a very low resistance as demonstrated by the end-to-end pressure drop measured at various blood flows. The Minifilter plus presents higher spontaneous filtration rates at a given blood flow. The

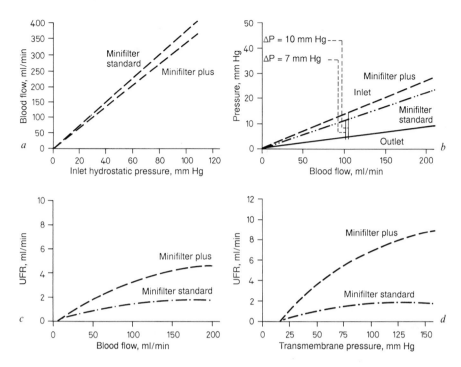

Fig. 1. Comparison of the two Minifilters (standard and plus) in terms of hydraulic characteristics. *a* Blood flow versus inlet hydrostatic pressure (venous pressure = 0). *b* Pressure profile inside the two filters at different blood flows. *c* Spontaneous UFRs of the two filters at different blood flows (venous pressure = 0, UF pressure neg. = 0). *d* UFR versus transmembrane pressure (blood flow fixed at 100 ml/min, K_f = 30 ml/h/mm Hg/m²).

ultrafiltration rate (UFR) is significantly higher in the Minifilter plus where 2–6 ml/min can be achieved. On the contrary, in the Minifilter standard, the curve reaches the plateau at about 2 ml/min. The operational parameters of in vivo application are reported in table 1. The operational parameters recorded in patient 16 are different because the Minifilter plus was utilized. It can be noted that, in comparison with the other cases treated with the Minifilter standard, blood and plasma flows were similar, while UFR was significantly higher. Despite the higher filtration fraction, the heparin requirement was not different and the filter operated for 4 days continuously without clotting problems or complications.

Discussion

CAVH and CAVHD in newborns represent not only an alternative to hemo- or peritoneal dialysis, but a real first-choice treatment for acute

Table 1. Operational parameters in the treated population

Patient No.	Blood flow ml/min	Plasma flow ml/min	UFR ml/min	Filtration fraction, %
1	28.0 ± 3.1	19.6 ± 2.6	1.1 ± 0.2	6.0 ± 1.3
2	25.2 ± 2.4	18.7 ± 2.0	1.0 ± 0.1	5.2 ± 0.1
3	15.4 ± 4.2	9.8 ± 3.9	0.8 ± 0.3	8.0 ± 1.6
4	22.0 ± 3.3	14.3 ± 3.0	0.7 ± 0.2	5.3 ± 1.0
5	31.3 ± 3.1	22.4 ± 2.9	1.0 ± 0.2	4.4 ± 0.9
6	21.5 ± 1.4	13.6 ± 0.9	0.9 ± 0.2	6.6 ± 0.7
7	19.4 ± 2.0	10.9 ± 1.2	0.9 ± 0.2	8.2 ± 0.6
8	24.6 ± 3.5	15.5 ± 2.1	0.8 ± 0.1	5.1 ± 0.5
9	33.1 ± 4.3	24.2 ± 3.0	0.9 ± 0.1	3.7 ± 1.1
10	35.0 ± 5.0	22.6 ± 3.1	1.1 ± 0.1	4.8 ± 1.3
11	19.1 ± 2.2	11.0 ± 1.1	0.7 ± 0.2	6.3 ± 0.2
12	27.9 ± 4.1	15.9 ± 1.9	0.9 ± 0.2	5.6 ± 0.3
13	13.2 ± 4.0	7.5 ± 1.5	0.5 ± 0.1	6.6 ± 0.5
14	28.2 ± 2.7	17.8 ± 1.6	1.0 ± 0.2	5.6 ± 0.4
15	31.7 ± 2.9	19.4 ± 1.3	0.8 ± 0.3	4.1 ± 1.3
16	36.6 ± 4.4	21.9 ± 2.8	2.9 ± 1.1	13.2 ± 1.2[a]

[a] Minifilter plus.

renal failure. The recent development of a new series of devices especially designed for this purpose permitted a definite improvement in the quality and efficiency of this treatment. This fact is further proved by a percentage of survival in our population of 43.75%. In all patients the correction of fluid imbalances, azotemia and acidosis was effective and the clinical tolerance to the therapy was excellent.

References

1   Ronco C: Continuous arteriovenous hemofiltration in infants; in Paganini EP (ed): Acute Continuous Renal Replacement Therapy. Den Haag, Nijhoff, 1986, p 201.
2   Ronco C, Brendolan A, Bragantini L, Fabris A, Feriani M, Chiaramonte S, Milan M, Dell Aquila R, La Greca G: Technical and clinical evaluation of a new polyamide hollow fiber for CAVH. Int J Artif Organs 1988;11:33–38.
3   Lauer A, Saccaggi A, Ronco C, Belledonne M, Glabman S, Bosch JP: Continuous arterio-venous hemofiltration in the critically ill patients. Ann Intern Med 1983;99:455–460.

Dr. Claudio Ronco, Department of Nephrology, St. Bortolo Hospital,
I-36100 Vicenza (Italy)

Sieberth HG, Mann H, Stummvoll HK (eds): Continuous Hemofiltration.
Contrib Nephrol. Basel, Karger, 1991, vol 93, pp 257–260

Continuous Arteriovenous Hemofiltration versus Continuous Venovenous Hemofiltration in Critically Ill Pediatric Patients

G. Zobel, E. Ring, M. Kuttnig, H.M. Grubbauer

Department of Pediatrics, University of Graz, Austria

Continuous arteriovenous hemofiltration (CAVH) for renal support allows the control of fluid balance and metabolic derangement in critically ill patients [1, 2]. However, in hypercatabolic states, azotemia cannot be controlled adequately by means of CAVH because of low urea clearance [3]. Continuous venovenous hemofiltration (CVVH) offers the advantage of higher urea clearance [4]. We report our experience with both treatment modes in 52 critically ill infants and children.

Patients and Methods

The clinical features of the patients are presented in table 1. Forty-seven patients (90%) were on mechanical ventilation and 44 (85%) needed vasopressor support. Indications for renal support were: acute renal failure (4); multiple organ system failure (44); severe metabolic disorders (2); diuretic-resistant hypervolemia (1), and severe hypernatremia (1).

Six different hemofilters were used. The extracorporeal filling volume during CAVH and CVVH ranged from 9 to 60 ml and from 36 to 120 ml, respectively. A roller pump (Gambro AK10™, Gambro, Hechingen, FRG) with exchangeable pump headings was used for CVVH. The blood flow of the pump ranged from 12 to 75 ml/min and from 50 to 300 ml/min, respectively. Anticoagulation for both treatment modes was achieved with heparin and/or prostacyclin. Fluid in- and output was balanced by a microprocessor-controlled fluid control system (Equaline, Amicon, Lexington, Mass., USA). Data are given as means $\pm$ SEM. Student's t test for unpaired samples and χ^2 test were used for comparison.

Results

The operational data of both treatment modes are presented in figure 1 and table 1. As shown in figure 2, a marked hemodynamic instability was observed in a critically ill infant during CVVH, whereas CAVH was well tolerated even by critically ill preterm and term infants. In children older than 1 year, only a slight fall of blood pressure was noticed immediately after starting CVVH. A femoral artery thrombosis occurred during CAVH and a thrombosis of the inferior vena cava during CVVH. Local bleeding due to brachial artery cannulation was observed in 2 infants. From the

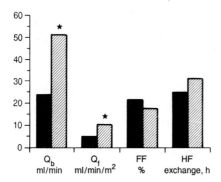

Fig. 1. Operational data during CAVH (■) and CVVH (▨). Q_b = Blood flow rate; Q_f = ultrafiltration rate; FF = filtration fraction; HF = hemofilter. *p < 0.01.

Table 1. Clinical features of critically ill infants and children with continuous renal support (n = 52; mean ± SEM)

	CAVH (n = 35)	CVVH (n = 17)
Age, years	4.03 ± 1.0	5.8 ± 1.6
Body weight, kg	16.2 ± 3.5	24.3 ± 6.3
Sex ratio, M/F	24/11	12/5
Duration of renal support, h	118.7 ± 19.9	115.2 ± 31.8
Serum creatinine, mg/dl		
Pretreatment	3.04 ± 0.48	2.5 ± 0.36
Posttreatment	2.2 ± 0.26	1.9 ± 0.2
Serum urea, mg/dl		
Pretreatment	126 ± 14.8	125.3 ± 22.3
Posttreatment	99 ± 8.3	83.6 ± 9.8
Urea clearance, ml/min/m²	5.1 ± 0.6	10.8 ± 1.4*
Outcome		
Survivors	21 (60%)	6 (35%)
Nonsurvivors	14 (40%)	11 (65%)

* p < 0.005.

technical point of view, there were some problems with continous blood flow during CVVH in small infants because of venous vessel wall aspiration when the catheter tip was located in the superior or inferior caval veins. CVVH ran without problems when the catheter tip was advanced to the right atrium in small infants or in children with a body weight above 12 kg.

The survival rate of the total group was 52%. Mortality rate in the CVVH group (65%) was higher than in the CAVH group (40%).

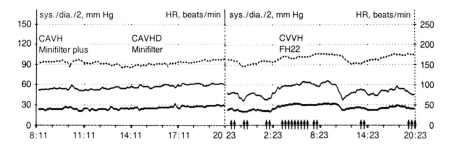

Fig. 2. Heart rate (HR; beats/min) and arterial pressure (mm Hg) in a neonate during CVVH, CAVH and arteriovenous hemodialysis (CAVHD).

Discussion

Usually azotemia can be controlled satisfactorily by means of CAVH in normocatabolic patients. However, in hypercatabolic patients serum creatinine and urea levels may increase during CAVH [3]. In order to improve urea clearance in critically ill patients with multiple organ system failure, continuous arteriovenous hemodialysis and CVVH have been recently introduced [4, 5]. In our infants and children azotemia was satisfactorily controlled with both treatment modes. Whereas hemodynamic stability was maintained during CAVH in all infants and children, CVVH was associated with a marked hemodynamic instability in small infants. Urea clearance was significantly higher during CVVH (p < 0.001). Using a double-lumen catheter CVVH was technically more difficult in small infants than CAVH. This problem can be overcome by using 2 single-lumen catheters and placing the suction catheter into the upper part of the right atrium.

In conclusion, CAVH and CVVH are effective methods of renal support in critically ill infants and children. CAVH provides hemodynamic stability whereas CVVH generates higher urea clearances and is associated with hemodynamic instability. Despite effective continuous renal support the mortality still remains high in children with multiple organ system failure.

References

1   Lauer A, Saccaggi A, Ronco C, Belledonne M, Glabman S, Bosch JB: Continuous arteriovenous hemofiltration in the critically ill patient. Ann Intern Med 1983;99:455–460.

2   Zobel G, Trop M, Ring E, Grubbauer HM: Arteriovenous hemofiltration in children with multiple organ system failure. Int J Artif Organs 1987;10:233–238.

3   Olbricht CJ: Continuous arteriovenous hemofiltration: The control of azotemia in acute renal failure; in Paganini EP (ed): Acute Continuous Renal Replacement Therapy. Boston, Nijhoff, 1986, pp 123–141.

4   Favre H, Levy M, Klohn M, Suter PM: Continous veno-venous hemofiltration; in
    Paganini EP (ed): Proc Third Int Symp on Acute Continuous Renal Replacement
    Therapy. Kidney Foundation, 1987, pp 87–93.
5   Dickson DM, Brown EA, Kox W: Continuous arteriovenous haemodialysis (CAVHD):
    A new method of complete renal replacement therapy in the critically ill patient.
    Intensive Care World 1988;5:78–80.

Gerfried Zobel, MD, Department of Pediatrics, University of Graz,
Auenbruggerplatz, A–8036 Graz (Austria)

Sieberth HG, Mann H, Stummvoll HK (eds): Continuous Hemofiltration.
Contrib Nephrol. Basel, Karger, 1991, vol 93, pp 261–263

Relationship between Erythropoietin and Trace Elements

Shinichi Hosokawa[a], *Atsushi Oyamaguchi*[a], *Osamu Yoshida*[b]

[a]Utano National Hospital and [b]Kyoto University Hospital, Kyoto, Japan

Erythropoietin was the first of the hemopoietic growth factors to be identified and so far the only one found to act as a true regulatory hormone. Production of this hormone, primarily by endothelial cells of the peritubular capillaries in the cortex and outer medulla of the kidney, is abrogated in most parenchymal renal diseases. Recently, recombinant DNA technology has allowed clinicians to bypass erythropoietin deficiency [1–3]. Stimulation of erythropoiesis by Epoetin Alfa (EP; Epogen, Amgen, Thousand Oaks, Calif., USA; Kirin, Sankyo, Tokyo, Japan; recombinant human erythropoietin) has allowed us to threat the anemia of patients on chronic hemodialysis. The success of EP therapy has conclusively demonstrated that erythropoietin deficiency is the major cause of the anemia of end-stage renal disease [4]. Here, we studied the relationship between EP and trace elements.

Materials and Method

Sixty-two patients with anemia undergoing chronic hemodialysis were randomly chosen and treated with EP. There were 34 males and 28 females, with an average age of 52 years. They underwent 3 times a week a 5-hour hemodialysis. Various kinds of dialyzers were used. At the start of EP treatment, average hematocrit (Hct) levels were 22%. EP (1,500 IU) was administered intravenously before the end of each hemodialysis; a total of 36,000 IU EP was given to all patients in 2 months. Hct levels increased significantly ($p < 0.01$) by 29.8% (average). Thereafter, an average of 1,500 IU EP was administered once a week, keeping on average 30% Hct levels for 3 months. Before the start of EP therapy and after the 5 months of EP therapy, serum aluminium (Al), silicone (Si), copper (Cu) and zinc (Zn) were measured with a Hitachi flameless atomic absorption spectrophotometer.

Sampling and storage of blood were performed free of contamination with trace elements. For statistical analysis, Student's t tests were used. $p < 0.05$ was considered as statistically significant.

Results

Serum Al levels decreased significantly (p < 0.01) from 24.4 ± 9.4 μg/dl before EP treatment to 18.4 ± 7.2 μg/dl after 5 months of EP treatment. Serum Si levels decreased also significantly (p < 0.01) from 62 ± 16 to 51 ± 8 μg/dl. However, serum Cu values were not significantly changed. Serum Zn levels increased significantly from 65 ± 18 to 74 ± 12 μg/dl.

Discussion

It is well known that serum Al levels [5] and serum Si values [6] are high in patients on chronic hemodialysis. Serum Zn levels are low in patients with chronic renal failure undergoing hemodialysis [7], while serum Cu levels are normal in patients on chronic hemodialysis. A potential disadvantage of correcting anemia by EP treatment might be a reduction of dialysis efficiency. In patients with a Hct greater than 40% a significant reduction of dialysis efficiency has been observed [8]. In general, serum iron levels decrease significantly with the increase in dosage of EP. Erythron transferrin uptake increases more than 3-fold under the stimulus of EP, and the consumption of available iron may lead to functional iron deficiency, which secondarily attenuates the response to the hormone. To avoid this, patients normally receive oral or intravenous iron supplementation before commencing EP treatment.

It is well known that serum Al and Si levels are high in patients on chronic hemodialysis. Recently, studies have indicated that a microcytic hypochronic anemia develops in dialyzed patients with high serum Al levels. Al overload dose indeed depress hematopoiesis in dialyzed patients, and the severity of the anemia and microcytosis depends on the degree of the Al overload. The mechanism of the anemia is due to a decrease in red-cell production. Al overload causes a reversible block in heme synthesis due to either a defect in porphyrin synthesis or impaired iron utilization.

Anemia was dramatically improved in the hemodialyzed patients treated with EP, indicating that serum Al levels decrease due to improvement of anemia in patients undergoing chronic hemodialysis. Serum Si levels significantly decreased with EP treatment, but this mechanism is unknown. Serum Cu values did not significantly change with EP treatment. Serum Zn levels increased significantly (p < 0.01) with EP treatment. These facts indicate that biological activities, including appetite, are augmented depending on the increase in Hct values. Because of an increase in appetite, serum Zn levels probably increase with EP treatment.

In conclusion Serum Al and Si levels decrease significantly (p < 0.01) with EP treatment, whereas serum Zn levels increase significantly (p < 0.01). These facts indicate good clinical effects of EP treatment. However, as these mechanisms are still unclear, further investigations are needed.

References

1   Winearls CG, Oliver DO, Pippard MJ, Reid C, Downing MR, Cotes PM: Effect of human erythropoietin from recombinant DNA on the anemia of patients maintained by chronic hemodialysis. Lancet 1986;ii:1175–1178.

2   Eschbach JW, Egrie JC, Downing MR, Browie JK, Adamson JW: Correction of anemia of end stage renal disease with recombinant human erythropoietin: Result of a phase I and II clinical trial. N Engl J Med 1987;310:73–78.

3   Casati S, Passerini P, Campise M: Benefits and risk of protracted treatment with human recombinant erythropoietin in patients having hemodialysis. Br Med J 1987;295:1017–1020.

4   Schaefer RM, Kuerner B, Zech M, Denninger G, Boeneff C, Heidland A: Treatment of the anemia of hemodialysis patients with recombinant human erythropoietin. J Artif Organs 1988;11:249–254.

5   Hosokawa S, Tomoyoshi T, Kawamura J, Yoshida O: Changes in serum aluminum concentration during hemodialysis. ASAIO J 1984;7:75–79.

6   Hosokawa S, Maeda T, Tomoyoshi T, Yoshida O: Silicon in chronic hemodialysis patients. ASAIO J 1987;10:260–264.

7   Hosokawa S, Tomoyoshi T, Yoshida O: Zinc transport during hemodialysis. Artif Organs 1986;10:30–36.

8   Shinaberger J, Miller JH, Gardner PW: Erythropoietin alert: Risk of high hematocrit hemodialysis. Trans ASAIO 1988;34:179–184.

Shinichi Hosokawa, MD, Utano National Hospital, 8 Ondoyama-cho,
Narutaki, Ukyo-ku, Kyoto-City 616 (Japan)

Sieberth HG, Mann H, Stummvoll HK (eds): Continuous Hemofiltration.
Contrib Nephrol. Basel, Karger, 1991, vol 93, pp 264–266

Stress-Induced Gastrointestinal Tract Hemorrhage Management by Continuous Hemofiltration: Gastrin Removal Evaluation

D. Journois, G.N. Francoual, D. Chanu, C. Drévillon, P.H. Cugneuc, D. Safran

Réanimation chirurgicale, Hôpital Laënnec, Paris, France

Stress-induced gastrointestinal tract hemorrhage (SIGH) is a frequent acute renal failure (ARF) complication severely affecting prognosis when it occurs [1]. Continuous hemofiltration (CHF), which is known to be an efficient and well-tolerated renal replacement method, is often used in these patients. This preliminary study, following a case report, was designed to assess what could be the contribution of CHF gastrin purification in SIGH treatment.

Case Report

An obese 62-year-old man was admitted for septic shock 2 days after having been operated on for large bowel occlusion. A septic state and prolonged low cardiac output syndrome were responsible for an ARF. Investigations revealed *Pseudomonas aeruginosa* pneumonia. Uremia was 72 mmol/l and bleeding time was increased (>8 min). Treatment included associated mechanical ventilation, antibiotics and correction of hemodynamic disorders, Gastric pH was kept above 5 using ranitidine infusion. Renal replacement was assumed by CHF. On day 4 of evolution, while the inotropic support was just discontinued, a severe gastric bleeding occurred requiring a mean rate of 8 packed red cells transfusion in 24 h. A wide gastroduodenal hemorrhagic area without any localized ulceration was found. Blood gastrin level (BGL) was 63 ng/l. Bleeding stopped after 52 h of CHF associated with intravenous omeprazole (120 mg/day), pirenzepine and sucralfate in cold water periodic topical infusion. Gastritis disappeared and the fibroscopic examination revealed a small easy-to-treat hemorrhagic ulcer on day 4. BGL was 8 ng/l and uremia 13 mmol/l at this time.

Material and Methods

Four more patients suffering from ARF treated with venovenous CHF (AN-69S Hospal® hemofilters) have been studied. Blood line thrombosis was prevented using a continuous infusion of a low molecular weight heparin (enoxaparin) at a dose of 1.2 mg/kg. The received intravenous ranitidine (2 mg/kg/day). (BGL) were radioimmunologically assayed in ultrafiltrate, arterial and venous lines at the onset of CHF, 24, 48 and 72 h later (CEA,

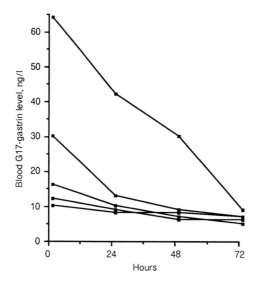

Fig. 1. Evolution of blood G17-gastrin level over time after onset of CHF in 5 patients.

Sorin, Biomedica, Saluggia, Italy). Sieving (S) and clearance (Cl) coefficients have been calculated using the rigorous formula of Colton-Henderson [2] which uses arterial (Ca), venous (Cv) then ultrafiltrate concentrations (Cu) and output rate (UFR): $S = 2 \times Cu/(Ca + Cv)$ and $Cl = Cu \times UFR/Ca$.

Results

Mean CHF blood flow was 95 ml/min. Ultrafiltration rate was 720 ± 110 ml/h. Observed BGL were within the normal range in 4 patients. Calculated clearance and sieving coefficients were respectively 8.1 ± 3.1 and 0.53 ± 0.14 ml/min. BGL evolution over time is reported in figure 1.

Discussion

Gastrointestinal bleeding and hypergastrinemia (a powerful gastric secretion activator) are commonly associated with uremia [3]. This is probably due to a reduced removal of gastrin by the kidney and/or an increased gastrin production resulting from an impairment of the negative feedback mechanism [3]. G17-gastrin molecular weight (about 2,100) explains its high CHF removal. Nonetheless, it is possible that removal per se may not have been responsible for SIGH ending in this patient: renal function replacement on the one hand, both nutritional and electrolyte balance on the other, may also be involved in CHF efficiency. Our results indicate that CHF might be an effective complement through substantial gastrin removal. However, CHF seems to be the optimal extrarenal purification method in these cases because BGL remains high during regular hemodialysis treatment [4]. Further studies should be undertaken to evaluate CHF in patients with hypergastrinemia and normal renal function.

References

1   Steinman P, Acute Renal Failure. Edinburgh, Churchill Livingstone, 1985 pp 723–262.
2   Kronfol NO, Lau AH, Colon-Rivera J, Libertin C: Trans Am Soc Intern Organs 1986; 32:85–87.
3   Muto S, Murayama N, Asano Y, Hosoda S, Miyata M: Hypergastrinemia and achlorhydria in chronic renal failure. Nephron 1985;40:143–148.
4   Owyang C, Miller LJ, DiMagno EP, Brennan LA Jr, Go VLW: Gastrointestinal hormone profile in renal insufficiency. Mayo Clin Proc 1979;54:769–773.

Dr. D. Journois, Réanimation chirurgicale, Hôpital Laënnec,
42, rue de Sèvres, F–75007 Paris (France)

Subject Index